T0107150

Praise for

DR. RASKIN AND ADVANCED DDS

"I have been using Advanced DDS for over thirty-two years. Dr. Raskin and his team are amazing. He has the latest and greatest, state-of-the-art equipment. They are all very professional, experienced and make you feel comfortable. We have referred many patients who have fears of dental work and all have said Advanced DDS made them comfortable and eliminated their fears."

PATIENT JOE P. (VALLEY STREAM, NY)

"Let me preface this review by saying that over the past twenty-six years, I have had a crippling fear of dentists. So bad that I had allowed my teeth to fall apart just to avoid having to go to the dentist. About a year ago, after not being to a dentist in over six years, the pain in my mouth became too much to handle. I was referred to Dr. Raskin. Skeptical, but in major pain, I decided to give him a shot. The work he did on me was extensive (once per week visits for over three months). Each time, Dr. Raskin made sure that I was comfortable and explained everything to me along the way. He went above and beyond to make sure I was calm and relaxed before starting any procedures and was extremely gentle throughout. The office is extremely clean and by far the most state-of-the-art I have seen, offering the best technology in the field. After being terrified of dentists for years Dr. Raskin has been the only one to get me past that. His office staff is extremely friendly and will not rush you like most other doctor's offices. I never waited at his office, they were always on top and most of the time even took me in early when I was ready. I strongly suggest Dr. Raskin—by far the best doctor I've ever been to."

PATIENT BLAKE C. (HUNTINGTON STATION, NY)

"FULL DISCLOSURE: I actually went to high school with Dr. Raskin, and after seeing his ads on television, I decided to give him a call and arrange an appointment. I have seen a handful of dentists over the years and have not really been totally satisfied and felt it was time for a change. The entire process, from my initial phone call to the appointment and the follow up, was a truly unique and positive experience. Not only did they text me to remind me for follow ups, but when you get to the office, there is virtually no paperwork—just about everything is done on a computer. The first thing that impressed me was the staff. After speaking with reception, I was invited to a tour of the office. At first I thought, "why do I need a tour of a dental office?" But after taking a tour with Haley I now understand. It was one of the most complete, professional and state-of-the-art dentist offices I have ever seen. From their in-house dental lab, 3-D imaging and even an in-house water treatment system, they have thought of everything. I was truly impressed."

PATIENT BILL S. (OLD BETHPAGE, NY)

"Love, love, love Advanced DDS. I'm here now and anxiety free. That's something I never thought I would ever say at a dentist's office. Best thing I ever did was make the decision to come here! Usually I go for a first appointment then fear going back. I don't have that problem with Advanced DDS. This is my third time here and it wasn't a planned visit. I got a call this morning that there was an open timeslot and I could come in today instead of waiting another week. I didn't even hesitate to say yes. Thank you to everyone at Advanced DDS for making me feel so comfortable!!!"

PATIENT GINA S. (MERRICK, NY

"Dentistry used to be up there as one of my greatest fears. In the past, I had a lot of pain with other dentists. Since I started going to Dr. Raskin at Advanced DDS, this has all changed. I have had many procedures done besides check-ups and cleanings such as treating cavities, crown removal and replacement, a wisdom tooth pulled with sedation, whitening, and veneers. I have not experienced any pain throughout any of this and was constantly checked on throughout the procedures to make sure I was doing ok. This office is big, clean, and full of all the most amazing, cutting edge technology. Another thing I would like to mention is the staff. I have never been in any doctor's office where everyone who works here is nice, friendly and patient. Not a trace of an attitude and always willing to help with whatever you may need. In addition, I have never had to wait more than five minutes to be called in. These things are a rare find in health care today. I can't recommend his doctor and this office enough."

PATIENT ROBYN W.

"A first-class experience from beginning to end. Always friendly service, nice amenities such as fresh cookies, apples and beverages. Dr. Raskin is up to date on all the latest developments in modern dentistry and knows how to help you relax during treatment. I highly recommend Advanced DDS."

PATIENT TRISH I.

"As always, Dr. Raskin and his staff go beyond what is expected to make a very stressful experience painless and stress free. I have been a patient of Dr. Raskin's for many years, and would not go anywhere else. He is professional, proficient and a pleasure to deal with. Five stars!"

PATIENT SUSAN F.

"Dr. Raskin has created a dental practice that far exceeds your expectations. I had put off seeing a dentist, but when I found Advanced DDS and went for a consultation, I was immediately put at ease by his staff. I highly recommend Dr. Raskin and look forward to many years of pain-free, anxiety-free treatment. One visit will convince you have made the right choice. I have also been treated by Dr. Thomas and was extremely satisfied with the experience. I wish them the best of luck in their beautiful new facility in Garden City."

PATIENT DEAN E.

"I've been a patient of Dr. Raskin for over ten years. Great practice. Starting with their punctuality. Don't recall ever waiting more than five minutes for my appointment (rare with any medical practice, in my experience). Office always has the newest technology and equipment. Beyond routine cleanings and fillings. I've needed a couple of crowns over the years and Dr. Raskin is an artist! Never had a problem with the work done. Highly recommended!"

PATIENT EDWARD R. (ROSLYN HEIGHTS, NY)

"I would highly recommend Dr. Raskin and his staff to anyone in need of dental work. I am having a wonderful experience and have no anxiety about completing my work. The procedure has been pain free and the results are looking wonderful. Recovery was quick."

PATIENT MARGUERITE N.

"I have always been scared of the dentist, but I needed a root canal/crown, and Advanced DDS made the experience painless and actually as comfortable as possible. Beautiful office and amazing staff. Looking forward to my next appointment."

PATIENT JESSIE F.

"Thank you Dr. Raskin and your staff for making my first visit your office the most comforting experience. From the moment I arrived, everyone on your staff was welcoming, encouraging and informative. There is no doubt in my mind that I will continue to receive the same great service and care in the future."

PATIENT RACHEL C.

"I was a patient of Dr. Raskin's father for fifty years. When he retired, I started going to Dr. Brian and thought nobody could be as good as his father. WRONG! Dr. Brian Raskin and his staff are wonderful. They not only are up to the minute as far as new technology, but they are all professional, yet gentle and caring. My dental experiences at Advanced DDS have been a pleasure (and that says a lot when going to the dentist). Thank you Dr. Brian Raskin and your entire staff for all you do to make "going to the dentist" enjoyable!"

PATIENT JANICE M.

"I always have a wonderful experience going to the dentist now that I found Dr. Raskin. I no longer fear or dread going and it is always pain-free! I wish I found him sooner, but at least now I have a dentist who truly cares about his patients and the work he does is perfect! I would highly recommend him to anyone!! Thank you Dr. Raskin :)"

PATIENT THERESA S.

Better

THAN BASIC

DR. BRIAN RASKIN

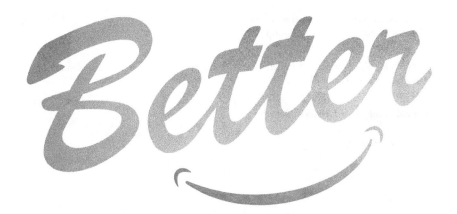

THAN BASIC

YOUR SMILE IS **WORTH THE BEST**

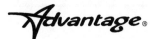

Copyright © 2018 by Brian Raskin.

All rights reserved. No part of this book may be used or reproduced in any manner whatsoever without prior written consent of the author, except as provided by the United States of America copyright law.

Published by Advantage, Charleston, South Carolina.
Member of Advantage Media Group.

ADVANTAGE is a registered trademark, and the Advantage colophon is a trademark of Advantage Media Group, Inc.

Printed in the United States of America.

10 9 8 7 6 5 4 3 2 1

ISBN: 978-1-59932-994-9
LCCN: 2018948456

Cover design by George Stevens.
Layout design by Carly Blake.

This publication is designed to provide accurate and authoritative information in regard to the subject matter covered. It is sold with the understanding that the publisher is not engaged in rendering legal, accounting, or other professional services. If legal advice or other expert assistance is required, the services of a competent professional person should be sought.

 Advantage Media Group is proud to be a part of the Tree Neutral® program. Tree Neutral offsets the number of trees consumed in the production and printing of this book by taking proactive steps such as planting trees in direct proportion to the number of trees used to print books. To learn more about Tree Neutral, please visit **www.treeneutral.com**.

Advantage Media Group is a publisher of business, self-improvement, and professional development books and online learning. We help entrepreneurs, business leaders, and professionals share their Stories, Passion, and Knowledge to help others Learn & Grow. Do you have a manuscript or book idea that you would like us to consider for publishing? Please visit **advantagefamily.com** or call **1.866.775.1696**.

*This book is dedicated to my father, Dr. Edward Raskin,
and my grandfather, Dr. William Raskin,
who started the Raskin family on a long tradition of
helping people improve their dental health.*

TABLE OF CONTENTS

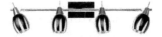

FOREWORD

Little did I know that my love of sailing would ultimately lead to my introduction to Dr. Brian Raskin. I met Dr. Raskin at The Knickerbocker Yacht Club in Port Washington, New York. We talked about our mutual love of sailing—it's a sport that allows you to become a part of nature for just a little while. You let the wind and water set your direction for the day. During that time, our families often went cruising together on the Long Island Sound. Sailing is a sport and an art. It involves skill and intuition, something Dr. Raskin also brings to his profession. During this time sailing, I discovered Dr. Raskin was a truly caring person, and this trait extended to his passion of dentistry as well.

Ultimately, I chose to see Dr. Raskin professionally as my dentist. When I first entered his office, I noted how remarkable it was—the front desk was friendly and welcoming, and I could tell Dr. Raskin's caring personality extended to his staff because they were extremely well-trained. The waiting rooms were clean and well appointed. There was attention to detail in common spaces that other offices did not consider important. The state-of-the-art technology was something I had never seen before at my previous dentist.

This attention to detail and incredible effort put into patient comfort was apparent in the treatment areas as well. They were as clean as you would expect—each examination chair had massage rollers, and each room had its own TV and stereo headphones.

Ever since we became friends through sailing, Dr. Raskin has been a trusted colleague. We have collaborated on many patients together and I have come to trust his opinion on complex cases. For example, we have coordinated care for sickly cardiovascular patients on multiple medications including antiplatelet agents following cardiac stents. We have also discussed treatment for patients on blood thinners/anticoagulants who also have atrial fibrillation. We no longer just discuss sailing. Our mutual love for our professions have allowed us to extend better care to our patients by sharing our knowledge and expertise.

I learn something new each time I interact with Dr. Raskin. I am pleased to have him as a friend and colleague. I know this book will enlighten some as to the differences you can find in the world of dentistry—you can see the differences as soon as you walk through his front door. His office has achieved a high quality of care through education and the addition of new technology. His office is the epitome of "better than basic." Throughout his career, he has strived to set himself apart from others by setting his bar for excellence always higher.

Dr. Jay Dubowsky
Board-Certified in Cardiology
Board-Certified in Internal Medicine
Practice in Manhasset, NY

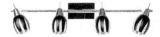

INTRODUCTION

Are you afraid to go to the dentist because of a bad experience you had as a child, or even as an adult? Do you know how to evaluate a dental office to determine whether it can deliver the care you need? Is your smile the best it can be? Do you know what insurance coverage really means?

Going to the dentist shouldn't be like confronting the boogeyman. With this book, I hope to show you how to choose a dentist, evaluate the level of care provided, and ease your fears about whether protecting your smile has to hurt. Getting proper care is worth it. After all, your smile is the first thing a stranger sees, and it contributes to your self-confidence and self-worth.

> With this book, I hope to show you how to choose a dentist, evaluate the level of care provided, and ease your fears about whether protecting your smile has to hurt.

I've been practicing dentistry for more than three decades and have built Advanced DDS in Garden City, Long Island, New York, into a premier practice, staffed by excellent doctors and staff who are equipped with the latest devices and materials. We are sensitive to our patients' needs and desires, and I want to share that experience and our expertise with you.

Dentistry's roots go back thousands of years, but recently there have been amazing strides made in technology. Let's face it. In more primitive times, dentistry hurt, as did most other medical procedures. When a doctor operated without anesthesia, the patient was told to bite the bullet. If the mouth needed work, however, biting said bullet wasn't an option. We've got much better ways of getting through procedures these days, involving not just local anesthetics but sedation at various levels. The patient's needs dictate what is used.

Check out your dentist's office. Is the carpet threadbare? Are there water spots on the ceiling? Is the wallpaper peeling? What about the equipment? Does it look like it came out of a Norman Rockwell painting, or is everything digital? Do you see the same dentist every time or does it seem like new people have joined the staff each visit? Is the doctor fresh out of dental school? Do you see evidence that the doctor takes continuing-education courses?

Dentistry need not hurt. Some 30 million to 40 million Americans admit to being fearful of going to the dentist.[1] They think they are alone and every procedure has to hurt. Wrong on both counts. Obviously, they're not alone. That's a pretty hefty number of people. With the use of local anesthetics, nitrous oxide, and various forms of sedation, patients can be kept comfortable throughout a procedure, whether it's a filling, a root canal, or an implant—in some cases, even a cleaning. The dentist just has to want to take the time to make sure the patient is sufficiently numb or sedated. And that goes for children, too. Even very young children should be taken to the dentist, and to help the experience be a positive one, they could be taken to a general dentist who is comfortable treating kids—or a pedodontist (a dentist who specializes working on children) like the ones who practice at

---

1   "What is Dental Anxiety and Phobia?" Colgate, https://www.colgate.com/
en-us/oral-health/basics/dental-visits/what-is-dental-anxiety-and-phobia

Advanced Children's Dentistry, our in-house children's dental office.

Children need to be treated differently than adults. Parents often let their fears rub off on their children before the children first set foot in a dentist's office. Don't scare your child. Children's teeth begin developing before birth and need to be taken care of when they first erupt. I'll explain some of the dos and don'ts that will help your children keep their teeth for a lifetime.

My practice has a relaxed atmosphere. We make our patients comfortable and don't rush people in and out. Many procedures that require multiple visits at other offices can be accomplished in just one visit to our office. We do our own modeling and milling on site, so some procedures that used to have a two-week lag between initiation and completion can be done in a less than a three-hour visit.

We also provide the little extras: drinks in the waiting room, comfortable seating, video games to distract the kids, music and television during procedures, patient-appreciation nights, and little raffles to put some fun into visits.

The insurance industry is trying to define dentistry as a commodity; nothing could be further from the truth. Everyone's needs are different, and your dentist has to be able to evaluate your mouth and develop a treatment plan that will allow you to keep your own teeth for as long as possible. That's my goal. I want my patients to keep what they were given during childhood for the rest of their lives. No denture, implant, or crown is better than a natural tooth.

Insurance just doesn't pay your dentist enough to cover the costs of excellent care, forcing some offices to cut corners on equipment, materials, and time spent with patients. You need to start thinking of dental insurance as a supplement that helps defray the costs of taking care of your teeth rather than a guarantee that you won't have to shell out anything extra.

Dentistry continues to evolve day-to-day, with constant innovations to new materials and techniques, and you want your dentist to be up to speed on all of them. Technology is not just the purview of the next smartphone or new-model vehicle. We're used to seeing new tech show up in the offices of medical doctors and at hospitals. It should be showing up in the dental office as well. Why fill a tray with gunk to take impressions when a digital scanner can produce a much more accurate result? An added benefit is that you no longer have to sit there while the gunk hardens, hoping the dentist won't mess it up on removal and be forced to do it all over again.

A healthy mouth is necessary for a healthy body, because bacteria from the mouth can migrate elsewhere, sometimes causing heart problems and even brain disorders. Not just the teeth, but the gums, soft tissue, and tongue must be kept healthy. Often a dentist can spot what hasn't yet become obvious to an internist.

You're not saving any money by avoiding the dentist. Just as not changing the oil in your car can lead to expensive repairs, not going to the dentist will cost thousands of dollars—better to perform routine maintenance than wait until disaster is looming. Don't think of it as expensive; think of it as an investment in yourself. And remember— putting off treatment means it will be that much more expensive to take care of a problem down the road.

If you think insurance is bewildering, you're right. One thing to remember is that the insurance company is not looking out for your best interests. It's interested mainly in maximizing profits for its investors. That means it will deny a claim whenever possible. If the claim is not denied, it might be delayed, repeatedly. The insurance company might say it can't find the claim or that it's incomplete. Bottom line is, you need to know what your insurance covers and doesn't cover—and then stay on top of the claims process.

The types of insurance policies out there are bewildering. In this book, I will explain the differences among DSOs, DMOs, DHMOs, PPOs, and independent/concierge practices. The level of care varies greatly. There are ten things you need to know about insurance, and I will explain them all.

Making your smile beautiful is not always costly. Whitening and straightening teeth may be all that's needed for you to regain your confidence. In other cases, veneers, crowns, or implants may be the answer. There's no reason to walk around with missing, decayed, or broken teeth. You'll be able to smile again.

I build trust with my patients. It's probably the most important thing I do. When I say treatment needs to be done, they can trust I'm telling them the truth. I don't recommend unnecessary procedures. I always have my patients' best interests at heart.

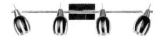

Chapter 1

TWENTY-FIRST CENTURY DENTISTRY

Dentistry has ancient roots and its development spanned the globe. The process was slow, with real progress not made until the twentieth century.

The ancient Sumerians identified "tooth worms" as the cause of decay in 5000 BC. The first dentist identified by name, however, was an Egyptian, Hesy-Ra, around 2600 BC. His tomb includes an inscription describing him as "the greatest of those who deal with teeth, and of physicians."

In ancient Greece, both Hippocrates and Aristotle wrote about tooth development and decay, but it wasn't until the Middle Ages that the Chinese started using "silver paste" to fill cavities (700 AD). By 1210, barbers were extracting teeth.

Dentistry became a serious profession in the 18th century, with the root canal gaining purchase by mid-century. In 1760, John Baker became the first medically trained dentist to immigrate to the United States. Fun fact: Paul Revere was a dentist.

John Greenwood invented the rotating drill in 1790 by rigging up the mechanism to the foot treadle from his mother's spinning wheel. The use of ether as an anesthetic for dental surgery was first tried in 1846, and Harvard established the first university-related dental program in 1867.

In 1903, the porcelain jacket crown was created and the "lost-wax" casting machine invented. Novocaine was introduced in 1905, the nylon toothbrush in 1938, and water fluoridation in 1945. Lasers came to the fore in 1960, the same year the first commercial electric toothbrush was marketed—and just two years after dentists started using the fully reclining dental chair.[2]

Dentists developed a negative reputation—in part due to the behavior of some, in part due to portrayals in books and movies. Who can forget Laurence Olivier (Szell) performing dental torture on Dustin Hoffman (Babe) in *Marathon Man* or Steve Martin's crazed character in *Little Shop of Horrors*? And let's not forget Peter Bonerz (Jerry) on the *Bob Newhart Show*—he was kind of a jerk and not very bright.

No wonder some people think dentists operate torture chambers.

The only sympathetic portrayal of a dentist I can think of was in *The Whole Nine Yards*, in which Matthew Perry (Nicholas "Oz" Oseransky) portrays a struggling dentist whose life is torn apart when famous gangster Jimmy "The Tulip" Tudeski (Bruce Willis) moves in next door, and Perry's character lets a notorious mob boss know.

MY EARLY YEARS

I grew up in a family of dentists. Dad was one. So was my grandfather. I toyed with being a physician early in my training—after all, doctors and dentists get the same basic training in their first two

---

2   "History of Dentistry Timeline," American Dental Association, last modified 2018, https://www.ada.org/en/about-the-ada/ada-history-and-presidents-of-the-ada/ada-history-of-dentistry-timeline.

years of school—but I ultimately opted to follow in Dad's and my grandfather's footsteps.

Their offices were typical for their times: x-ray machines, drills, cuspidor—exactly what you'd expect. Their record keeping was done with a pencil and a typewriter. Dad's office was in our home for at least thirty years. It was on the main floor and had a separate entrance.

Once I finished my training, I did a year-long general practice residency at Booth Memorial Hospital in Flushing, New York and then worked in two offices on Long Island. I hated that. Mondays, Wednesdays, and Saturdays, I was in office "A"; Tuesdays and Thursdays, I was in office "B." There were days I woke up not knowing where I was supposed to be.

Office "A" was also my first experience with HMO dentistry. It was an office that had many capitation plans and was as basic a dental practice as you could get. The walls were paneled. Equipment was in poor condition, and the staff was far from helpful. There were limited supplies, and the quality of the labs left much to be desired, but it was a good place for me to start. Remember, this was in the 1980s when insurance had just started making inroads into my profession. There were several dentists just like me who were also just out of school. The turnover at this office was significant. As soon as one dentist had enough and left, another new doctor would be hired to fill the spot. It was unusual for the patients to see the same doctor each visit. The assistants were as transient as the doctors. They also didn't care much about the patients. I worked two evenings until 9 o'clock. At about 8 p.m., my dental assistant would leave my room, and I would have to treat my patients solo. The assistants were busy closing the office so they could leave, which seemed to take precedence over the patients.

I very quickly discovered what type of dental practice I *didn't* want to work in or own. The office got paid by the insurance company based on the number of people who signed up. There was no incentive to treat these patients with any type of comprehensive dentistry. Extractions, dentures, and fillings were the mainstays, or as I call it, basic dentistry. I didn't last long there due to my frustration with the office and the low quality of care. I came from a family of dentists; I needed to do better than provide insurance-level dentistry. But more on that later. Let's go to office "B."

Office "B" was a fee-for-service office out on Long Island. It was owned by a single dentist who was also a nice guy. We seemed to hit it off from the beginning. He had a friendly patient base and a nice staff. I worked there for about eight months and was able to do quality dentistry without limiting my care to the demands of insurance. My patients appreciated their care and it was the total opposite from office "A." As time went on, though, I became restless. I never liked working for somebody else. From when I was a camp counselor at Fidel Country Day Camp, I always resented taking orders from others. I am sure that is why I own my own practice now. Having no boss to answer to is the only way I am happy. There was a possibility of a partnership with the practice or, so I was told, there might be when I was hired. We were drawing up plans for a new office in a condominium office complex across the street and started drafting a partnership agreement. My wife and I were already thinking about moving out on Long Island near the office. But a few months later, the owner got cold feet and wasn't willing to pull the trigger on any of our plans. I'm not good at waiting things out to see what is going to happen. I have always been a doer—and it was time to do.

In 1984, I went out on my own.

My first office was in the basement of a home. Not mine, though. It was in the basement of the home belonging to the widow of a deceased dentist in Valley Stream, New York., from whom I bought the practice for $69,000—including all 75–100 patients and a fully equipped office, such as it was. I had heard about the practice from Dad, who'd heard about it from a colleague at a meeting.

This type of transition from academics to the real world was, at the time, very common. Even though I was coming right out of a general-practice residency, I was still very green. Dentistry is a complicated profession. It's kind of like skiing—a sport I love and have become very good at over time. A beginner can make it down the bunny run just fine, but going straight to double-black runs takes a lot of experience. Here, I was still on the bunny run of dentistry. I needed more practice, and what better way to do it than in someone else's office?

It was strange being in someone else's home, but there was a separate entrance, so patients didn't have to walk through the kitchen or living room.

The office was in a brick split-level, but it hadn't been updated in a long time. The walls were paneled or had flocked wallpaper (you know the kind, red with a paisley design), and the floors were covered in linoleum. The equipment was old, probably dating back to the 1950s. The machines were bright yellow and looked like elaborate fire hydrants made for torture. The drill had belts that moved around and around. The air compressors and suction units were astonishingly loud—so loud, in fact, that if you closed your eyes, you could imagine yourself in a machine shop or garage. The x-ray machine was on a mechanical timer, which made it more difficult to control the amount of radiation given to a patient. The windows were high up. Patients could only look out into the shrubs. One of the treatment rooms housed the sewage-cleanout trap. We had one phone line, one person at the front desk, and a typewriter I had received for my bar-mitzvah. My private office was so small I had to build a desk specifically for the room to make it fit.

The environment didn't instill confidence, let alone fond memories. It definitely was not a relaxing setting for the patient. But it was a place I could start in. It worked—sort of.

After a while, I decided to update the décor. That upset my landlady, who thought the place looked just wonderful. I painted the paneling a light color, changed the wallpaper, added carpeting, and bought new equipment. I even hired a hygienist. I had three staff members in all: a receptionist, an assistant, and a hygienist. I was really cooking. Before my first son was born, my wife filled in at the desk. Little did she know that later on, after the kids were grown, she would be office manager of a group dental practice with a staff of twenty-eight. She had worked for her farther in the textile business before we started our practice. For the first week, she'd habitually answer the phones with: "Yarnell Fabrics." As you would guess, that didn't go over very well.

At first, I wasn't all that busy. This was also when video games were just coming out. Atari was my system of choice, and I spent a lot of time playing "Space Invaders" and "Missile Command." My wife would call and hear bing, bing, bing, bing, bing. She knew what I was doing.

I spent five years in that basement, slowly building my patient portfolio through direct mail and word of mouth. That same Atari computer on which I played "Space Invaders" also worked as a great word processor. I would churn out letters all day, inviting neighbors to come to my practice. Every week I would get one or two new patients who would help build my clientele so I could get out of the basement. You won't see many home offices now, and they won't exist at all eventually because of the way the dental business is changing, but we'll get into that later.

PHASE TWO

After five years, I decided it was time to move. I found a new building in Valley Stream. I needed $150,000 to build my new office, but the bank refused to loan me the money because I didn't have enough of a history or cash flow. The banker suggested just opening an office in the basement of my home. I asked him why he didn't put the bank in the basement of his home; he didn't have a response to that. To this day, I won't do business with that bank.

So instead of a loan, I went to a leasing company and ended up paying top dollar for the money I needed.

Looking back, I realize I set up that whole office for the cost of the CT scanner I bought for my current facility. Times have changed. Dentistry has become a very technology-intensive business. When I started out, the most expensive piece of equipment was an x-ray machine. When I purchased my first new x-ray machine, it was $2,500, and I took a five-year loan for it. Now, $2,500 does not even cover one electric drill.

My new office in Valley Stream was ultramodern. It was beautiful. I stayed in it for ten years. Along the way, I brought in another dentist who was considering retirement, and it was during this time I named my practice *Advanced DDS*. Because of all the technology I had in the office, he stayed far longer than he expected. Most dentists don't invest much into their practices at the end of their careers. Economically, it does not make sense. Equipment and technology are expensive, so if you are only going to be in practice for three to five more years, the return on the investment is just not there. For this reason, you often can tell when a practitioner is slowing down. This is one of the advantages of a group practice. There might be an older doctor who is slowing down, but there is always a younger doctor who needs the newest and the best. My associate stayed for more than five years.

Eventually, I had outgrown the space and was tired of paying rent, so it was time to move once again.

My third office, still in Valley Stream, was in a building I had purchased with another dentist, but we had separate practices. I hired several dentists before finding one who was going to stay. Across the street was another dentist. He was an older fellow, in his eighties. I was in my forties at the time. He was talking about slowing down, so I invited him to move in with me; I'd take care of all his administrative needs, and when he was ready to retire, his patients would be in good hands.

When I visited his office, I was appalled; it looked like the basement practice I had purchased fifteen years earlier. He was still taking impressions with an outdated technique that's not very accurate. It was barbaric in my eyes. He even had a typewriter he'd probably received for his bar-mitzvah, and his metal desk seemed right out of the Army surplus store.

That's when I realized that the appearance of the dentist's office can tell patients a lot about the quality of services they'll be getting. His attitude was: "It works. Why change?"

It's like my father saying, "My pencil works. What do I need a computer for?" (Dad now uses a computer and an iPhone, and probably wouldn't admit to ever saying that.)

But that dentist's attitude still is common among dentists. They're reluctant to buy new equipment because it's expensive. They don't want to learn new techniques because the old ones are good enough. The mentality is, "Why should I bother if I don't have to?" With insurance reimbursements no higher than they used to be, they don't have the money to spend on new equipment anyway. They don't even have the money to paint and buy new carpeting.

I met a guy recently who said he doesn't do anything with digital equipment, because he doesn't feel like learning anything new. I don't get an attitude like that! We're not plumbers. If you go into this profession, you should be required to stay up-to-date. You should be obligated to do the right thing. But, sadly, there is no obligation, and I see quality getting worse. Just recently, Mike came into my office with his dad for a second opinion. He's seventeen years old. His doctor had said the boy had a few cavities. Dad was a little suspicious and wanted me to check it out. He had taken photos with his iPhone of the x-rays and sent them to my office. The x-rays were the old film type. Now, I am not saying that film is bad, but I have not used film in my practice since my very early years. There are multiple advantages to digital x-rays. One is the lower radiation dose. There's also the ability to enhance the images and view them larger on a monitor. Again, film is not bad—but where has this guy been, and why hasn't he embraced a technology that has been around since 1998?

In my early days of dental school, doctors didn't wear gloves or worry about transmitting diseases to patients or even themselves. Instruments were sterilized between patients but drills were not; they were just wiped down with a disinfectant between patients. It was not very effective. Then the AIDS epidemic started and things changed. Universal protocols or precautions were established to protect the doctor and patient from disease. Even now, however, some dentists don't sterilize their drills between patients despite best-practices requirements. They don't follow the accepted protocols. If they can't afford to buy new wallpaper, they can't afford to buy the extra handpiece (drill) necessary for autoclaving between patients. You wouldn't believe how many of my assistants, who temp in other dentists' offices, have told me that. In one case, a dentist ran out of sterilized instruments and told the assistant to just wipe some down with disinfectant wipes. Ask your dentist if the drills are sterilized between patients or just once at the end of the day. If the latter is the case, make sure you're the first appointment of the day.

RECENT CHANGES

In recent years, technology has really changed. The first breakthrough was new materials for bonding: tooth-colored material that could be used to repair chips. The only problem was that at first, only one color—dubbed universal—was available. Compared to what's available now, we were still in the dark ages. People's teeth are not universally the same color. When I started out, I wasn't doing things much differently than my dad had three decades earlier, or even my grandfather. People went to the dentist expecting the worst—for good reason. They dreaded the needle used to inject novocaine. When my grandfather was in practice in the 1950s, the needle was used, boiled, then reused. No wonder it hurt! Now, needles are used once and are exceedingly sharp to reduce the pain of injection.

Sometimes, the anesthetic wouldn't actually work, and the patient would be in pain anyway. The materials tasted bad and smelled worse. And forget the music playing in the background; no one liked it. If we played classical, somebody would complain. Switch to rock, and older patients started to complain. Elevator music was universal, but nobody was happy. Eventually, I resorted to headphones and tapes. That way, everyone could be happy—at least with the music. Now we have televisions in every room with Netflix, Pandora, and cable channels. You can sit down and choose your music or favorite show. Each room can be different, but I find most people like the HGTV network. I'm not sure why, but everybody seems to like seeing homes being worked on. I guess everyone has dream houses.

Some dentists just don't care. Others actually seem to be sadists. While I was still in dental school, I observed at an emergency clinic.

I was watching one dentist work on a patient in his twenties, and he was hurting the poor kid. I was cringing. "What's wrong with this picture?" I asked myself. The dentist was doing what he had to do, and didn't care about hurting the patient. I said to myself, "I'm never doing that. That's not the way I'm going to work." I still vividly remember this thirty-eight years later, and I have made sure not to follow in that dentist's footsteps. It was probably a good experience for me. Instead of teaching me how to do something, it taught me how not to do something—ever.

And I don't. My current office in Garden City, Long Island, opened in 2013. Advanced DDS has twelve chairs and twelve treatment rooms, two of which are designed for children. I've got a pediatric dentist and five other doctors here including me. There is an oral surgeon who comes in once a week, plus four hygienists. And we do almost everything here. Three of us are trained in intravenous, or IV, sedation. The only thing we really send out is orthodontics for children.

All my doctors have at least five years of experience. I don't hire new graduates—even though some patients think those with newly acquired sheepskins are up-to-date on all the latest techniques. That's just wrong, however. New grads don't know much more than the basics, because that is all they are taught. There is a tremendous amount of information given during dental training. It's impossible to cover more than the basics. It takes at least five more years to really know what you're doing. New dentists are great for basics, but comprehensive treatments need specific expertise that can be acquired only over time. Either you go to specialty training after dental school or take continuing education courses until you have developed the skills to tackle complicated treatments.

I appreciate my patients and believe in giving back. In fact, we have various patient-appreciation events, including raffles. Recently,

I rented out a movie theater and filled it with 150 patients and their kids to watch *Thor*. We've raffled off trips to Mexico and given away American Express gift cards, barbecues, iPads, and TVs.

If you are local, please come to Advanced DDS. Sit back and relax, and be assured there's nothing to fear. If not, at least this book will help you learn about what to look for in a dentist and be better educated when choosing one in your area. This way you will be getting the best possible care—virtually pain free.

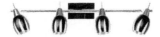

Chapter 2

FEAR FACTOR: GOING TO THE DENTIST DOESN'T HAVE TO HURT

There are two types of people who avoid going to the dentist: Those who don't really care about their teeth, and those who have had bad experiences and are afraid. In some cases, among the first group, people may look at dental care as too costly. In other cases, they may have other priorities, preferring to spend their money on fancy cars and elaborate vacations or cosmetic procedures like liposuction and breast augmentation. They figure, "Why fix a back tooth no one can see?" Their parents lost their teeth in their forties and wore dentures, and their grandparents wore dentures, so they expect to do so as well. Why invest in their mouths? We can't help people if they're not interested.

Not too long ago, Advanced DDS conducted a focus group. I wanted to find out what people liked about our office, why they came in for treatment, and why they did or did not follow through with the suggested course of action. I was interested in making the experience as good as it could be for my patients and wanted to know what people wanted. The results were very enlightening. There was a group that cared only about cost—but not because they didn't have the money. Some of them went on vacations, bought BMWs, or had cosmetic surgery. To them, their teeth were not important enough to spend any additional money on other than what their insurance allowed. It was about priorities. I decided that these people were not the type of patients we could work with at Advanced DDS.

The other group was made up of people who put their overall health and their dental health above—or at least on a par with—things like vacations and toys. This group appreciated the technology and the extra training our doctors have. They understood their teeth were important, even the ones in the back. They were willing to spend a little more for the peace of mind and quality they get at our office. This is the type of person we see at Advanced DDS. I am telling you this for one reason: To help you determine the kind of patient you are. What are your priorities and expectations? This plays a role in the type of dental office that will make you happy. Patients vary wildly—some are extremely comfortable and talkative, and others may have extreme anxiety and dental fear. I tend to see the latter quite often.

One of the reasons patients develop fears is because of the experiences they had as children. Their parents likely took them to dentists who didn't really want to handle children or didn't know how. They weren't pediatric dentists. Some would use size to intimidate the child or strap a child down to get the work done. This is especially true of children who were brought to clinics that weren't really set up for kids. Other children get their anxiety from parents who say things like, "This won't hurt—much." What are they thinking? They're planting the seed that dental work has to hurt, when in reality, going to the dentist should never hurt at all.

Or perhaps the fearful patient had a bad experience later in life where a dentist didn't wait for the anesthetic to work, or the anesthetic wore off midway through a procedure or treatment and the dentist didn't give any more.

We don't operate that way.

First, you can walk in and relax. The practice a safe place where you can wait in comfortable chairs. We don't throw people immediately into a dental chair. Instead, there's a consultation room where we can talk about your dental problems and how they can be approached. Then we conduct an examination and take X-rays. From that point, we can talk about specific procedures and decide whether or how to proceed. There are even television screens available for watching a movie while work on your mouth is being done.

Not everyone who walks through our doors becomes a regular patient. Though nearly all agree they like the appearance of our facilities, admire the technology we employ, and like our staff and amenities, some see the little extras as adding to costs. The can of seltzer in the waiting room is about 25 cents. Some patients think it poses an unnecessary cost while others appreciate the gesture. As I have said before, the only way some patients will do something is if it is covered by insurance.

THE FEAR FACTOR

Like I mentioned previously, patients come into the practice with dental fear all the time. Luckily, I know just what to do when it comes to the fearful patient. Fear of the dentist is like any other fear. Some people can't get on an airplane because of fear. Some can't climb up a ladder. Some can't leave their apartments. And some are too afraid to go to the dentist. It's a very real fear—it has two different names: *odontophobia* or *dentophobia*.

If you have a problem with your foot, it can be draped so you can't see what the doctor is doing or you can watch from a distance.

With your mouth, the dentist is right in your face, invading your personal space. I think this is one of the reasons that some people fear the dentist. We get into their space, and they can't get away—it can be claustrophobic to some.

Margaret walked into the office the other day. She's in her eighties and hadn't been to the dentist in years. She had a bad experience when she was just five or six years old—seventy-five years earlier. She went on and on about how the dentist hurt her. He wouldn't stop drilling. From that point on and for the next sixty-seven years Margaret hated the idea of going to the dentist and avoided it at any cost. This is a perfect example of how a single experience can affect patients' dental health for the rest of their lives. Margaret eventually became a great dental patient and after a few visits, she realized that dentistry had changed over the years. She is now able to go for her routine visits without any fear.

Another patient, Louise, came in with pain in her lower right jaw. She hadn't been to the dentist for years, but the pain was finally too much. After seeing our commercial for sedation dentistry, she decided that was the only way she was going to get the work done. When she came in, we took her into the conference room to explain how we do things—you don't want a fearful patient in a dental chair. She was crying and shaking. Her blood pressure was through the roof, and I hadn't even done anything yet. We told her we just were going to do an examination and take some x-rays. It wouldn't hurt. We decided she needed two crowns and a root canal, so we scheduled a two-hour sedation appointment for the work. The day of the appointment, she came in early with her husband and apologized for being a "bad" patient. She was shaking. Her doctor had prescribed sedatives, but they didn't do anything to curb her anxiety. My front desk warned me I'd better get started soon, because she was shaking and crying in the waiting room. To overcome that kind of fear, the dentist needs to create an atmosphere of trust.

Before taking her in for treatment, we comforted her, acknowledged her fears, and showed compassion. We were not just taking care of a root canal or whatever other work needed to be done. We were taking care of the *patient*, respecting her fear.

We don't just treat teeth. We change people's lives; treating teeth is just how we do it.

> **We don't just treat teeth. We change people's lives; treating teeth is just how we do it.**

So, we did the work and at the end of her appointment, Louise was amazed we were done and gave us a big smile. The next day she called the front desk to make sure we knew how wonderful her experience had been and to thank me. How often does a patient call a dentist the next day and say thank you?

Another example: Richard. He was what I call a dental invalid. His mouth was a mess. He's in his forties and never took care of his teeth. But he married a longtime patient who had been coming to me since she was a little girl, and she convinced him it was time to get his teeth fixed. His whole lower arch was shot. He was unable to go to restaurants because he couldn't chew in public. He covered his mouth and teeth with his hand because he was ashamed of the way they looked. He never smiled.

When we got him into the office for basic dentistry, we restored his upper teeth without sedation and decided to put implants on the bottom after removing those teeth. To put Richard at ease, we suggested sedation dentistry for the long surgical visit. Richard did well with the surgery and didn't remember a thing. That's the advantage of sedation. The whole process took four or five months, start to finish. The next time he came in for a routine cleaning, he pulled me over by the arm to thank me. He said that, though it was expensive, it was the best thing he ever had done for himself. It changed his life and how he felt about himself.

We used sedation on both those patients to alleviate their fears. When we do such procedures, there are always three of us in the room: the doctor, an assistant, and someone to record and watch the monitors. I'll talk about sedation dentistry in-depth in chapter five, but these are several types of sedation:

- **Minimal sedation** in which the patient is awake but relaxed

- **Moderate sedation** or **conscious sedation** in which the patient may slur words when speaking and not remember the procedure

- **Deep sedation** in which the patient is on the edge of consciousness but still can be awakened

- **General anesthesia** in which a patient is completely unconscious (we don't do this in the office unless an anesthesiologist is present)

We'll get into more detail on what's involved in each of these sedation methods in chapter five.

Advanced DDS has three dentists certified to administer IV sedation. Before I got my certification decades ago, I would call an anesthesiologist who would do the sedation, and I'd do the implants. The fees I had to charge were much higher as a result. It was also an inconvenience for the office and the patient. Our office is now fully set up for sedation. It is routine in our practice and the doctors and staff can set it up at a moment's notice.

I did my IV sedation training at Montefiore Medical Center in the Bronx, and I was certified by the state so that I could do my procedures without calling in another doctor. Initially, I just used it for implants, but it dawned on me that some patients wanted it for root canals and crowns as well. Some even wanted it for cleanings. So, we started offering sedation for all types of general dentistry as well as surgery. Very few dentists do that.

All my doctors are certified with advanced cardiac life support in case of an emergency—and an emergency can arise at any time, not just when sedation is involved. We have to maintain our certificates and, as a result, can handle the majority of things that can happen. You can have an emergency even with something as simple as a filling. Every dentist should be trained to handle emergencies. The most common emergency in a dental office is a person having a heart attack. Your doctors should be prepared.

THE HUMAN TOUCH

Not every dental office is equipped to do the kind of work we do. Part of that is dictated by economics, since insurance doesn't pay very well. The model means a lot of people need to be treated quickly to generate the revenue necessary to pay the bills. The dentist doesn't have the time to make sure a patient is numb and comfortable—nor does he or she care. It's not a priority.

Lower fees and higher volume may make sense for a mechanic, but it doesn't make sense when you're working on people. You give up the personal touch. A lot of these dental-maintenance organizations give dentists a specific amount of time to do a procedure. If it takes longer, the dentist is penalized. Requirements such as these are turning dental treatment into a commodity. Telling people to come to a particular office because it's cheaper—or because it's free—is sending the wrong message.

I have had insurance companies send letters to my patients,

telling them to go to a participating dental office to save money. They don't say that the office is as well qualified; they don't say the doctors have the same training; nor do they say that they will propose the best treatment. They just say it's cheaper. And as I keep on saying, cheaper is not better.

Some patients need hand-holding. Sometimes the doctor needs to talk to a patient to alleviate fears. I see a lot of patients who have been going to cheaper practices, and they're tired of it. They don't like the long waits or being treated like numbers. They don't like going back multiple times for the same thing. Time is increasingly valuable. Missing multiple days of work could cost more than the dentistry itself. These patients end up in my office.

There's an art to knowing how to keep a patient comfortable. I've had patients tell me they never got numb at a basic dentist's office. I have different ways of making patients comfortable. There are different types of anesthetic and different types of ways to administer these agents. Once they are comfortable, they then tell me they can't believe it didn't hurt.

The fearful patient finally decides to go to the dentist when mouth pain exceeds the pain of being afraid. Fearful patients think they're alone, that no one else shares their anxiety. When they find out they have plenty of company, they're happy! They find out about us after seeing a commercial or by doing an internet search or from a friend. They can't believe they've found us and want to know why more dentists don't approach treatment the way we do.

Now they're going to the dentist because they have a way to deal with their problems. Making that first phone call is the hardest part of the process.

The first thing we do with a new patient is build trust. We treat the person, not just the person's teeth. We bring patients into a conference room with a couch and comfortable chairs where they fill out a medical history form on a computer. Then an assistant comes in to talk about the patient's fears and what needs to be accomplished. After that, the doctor is invited in and the discussion continues. We talk about what brought the patient in and the patient's expectations. We explain what we do. Only after all that is a patient brought into a treatment room for an exam and x-rays.

All dental offices should operate this way to help the patient reframe the experience and learn to think differently about going to the dentist. Once you build that trust, you can get to the next step comfortably. Not every new patient needs or wants sedation; they just need the reassurance that it's there if they do want it. I don't hurt my patients. I know if I hurt them, they won't come back.

After the exam, we again retreat to the conference room to talk about what needs to be done. If they have dental anxiety, we discuss the various forms of sedation and figure out a plan—something simple first, then we build from there.

The majority of fearful patients just need reassurance they will be comfortable. Only about 15 to 20 percent of the practice involves sedation, and of those who begin with sedation, about half say they don't need it when they come in for the second or third time.

I had a patient, Walter, who needed his whole upper arch restored and demanded sedation. He wouldn't do anything without it. Two visits later, we were doing something that wasn't all that complicated, so he decided to try it without sedation. We had developed trust. After that, he never asked for sedation again. He needed those first two visits to develop trust and become comfortable in the dental chair. He would never have started treatment without sedation.

I mentioned the four types of sedation earlier: minimal, moderate, deep, and general anesthesia. The American Dental

Association recognizes that local anesthesia, sedation, and general anesthesia are an integral part of dentistry, for children as well as adults. Advanced DDS treats just adults, but Advanced Children's Dentistry treats the kids. At Advanced Children's Dentistry, we have a pediatric dentist who specializes in keeping children as comfortable as possible. We don't want them to develop the fears their parents might have had as kids.

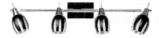

Chapter 3

WHY YOU SHOULD THINK CAREFULLY WHEN CHOOSING A DENTIST

The old adage, "You get what you pay for," is just as true in dentistry as anywhere else. Cut-rate prices can mean cut-rate materials. "Free" very often costs you more than you bargained for. Questionable advice does not have much value. That free item you're often promised when buying a product often is useless or of such poor quality that it breaks the first time you use it.

Think about that.

Do you really want that for your teeth? Your smile creates a first impression and contributes to your self-confidence.

Since the insurance industry got involved in dentistry, some people have started thinking of dentistry as a commodity, a sort of one-size-fits-all service where minimal treatment is good enough. One thing I have learned is that "good enough" seldom is good enough. Insurers pay dentists between 25 and 80 percent of what a service is worth. Eighty percent isn't so bad but 25 percent? The other 75 percent has to be made up somewhere, whether it is in upkeep of the office, the equipment and materials used, or the time a dentist actually spends with a patient. If you're looking for an office that's cheap, don't expect the same quality of service or treatments that you can get from a full-service dental office.

A friend of mine is an accountant, and he has three clients who are dentists. The three no longer can afford to run their offices because they don't take in enough money to cover overhead. Their solution is to get jobs working for someone else. Years ago, all three decided to accept insurance clients—both private insurance and government programs—to help fill in their schedules since they weren't that busy and hadn't been getting that many new patients. They figured they'd treat patients instead of sitting around, knowing they'd make less money but their time would be occupied.

They apparently weren't very good businessmen. Sure, they were busier and happy the insurance plans were sending them patients—but over the years they found there was no extra money for painting the walls or changing the carpeting. And if there isn't money for the cosmetics, think about what else there is no money for: new equipment, top-grade materials, the ability to provide proper—not just basic—care. In short, no money to upgrade the practice or really give patients the attention they need.

Dentistry, like anything else, is a business. Staff and rent need to be paid, supplies need to be purchased. To keep the business going, dentists in thrall to the insurance companies need to cut corners to make a living. They do this by buying cheaper materials, going on eBay or other sites, and ending up with expired materials, knockoffs, or other substandard materials masquerading as the real thing. They also send their lab work overseas where standards are not the same as in the United States.

Others might not be cleaning their instruments as well as they should. Like I mentioned before, between patients, drills and other equipment used need to be sterilized. The sterilization cycle takes time.

To properly sterilize dental instruments and drills, they need to be placed in an autoclave, a container that uses steam sterilization. This cycle should be between fifteen to thirty minutes at 270 degrees. Dental offices should also be testing their equipment with biological monitors. This method confirms that the equipment is working properly. Because the process is somewhat tedious—albeit, necessary—that means more equipment needs to be available to the practice. If a dentist can't afford to buy that extra equipment, that might mean just wiping down drills with disinfectant rather than sterilizing. And then there are the saliva ejectors, or "Mr. Thirsty," as some of the children call it, the plastic tubes that take the spit out of your mouth. Those are only supposed to be used once and then tossed, yet some offices use them more than once or cut them in half so they have two instead of one. Is that good enough for something going into your mouth?

If a dentist is getting only 25 to 80 percent of the regular fee, then the service is only going to be 25 to 80 percent of what it could be. You're not getting full service. There are some patients where a fifteen-minute cleaning is sufficient. There are others where multiple visits are necessary to bring their teeth and gums back to health. Which one are you? It is vital for a patient to ask whether the dentist is using a lab that meets US standards or if the work is being sent overseas where there is no quality control—whether implants are brand name or no name can save money for the dentist, but will be detrimental to your health. What about the experience of the dentists on staff? How long have they been in practice? At the same time, experience isn't everything. As I mentioned earlier, older dentists nearing retirement may be unwilling to invest in the latest equipment. Dentistry is not a commodity. Offices provide a different level of care depending on their expertise, values and conscience. You need to decide what your health and teeth are worth to you.

GETTING WHAT YOU PAY FOR

Some of my patients had been going to other dentists regularly, getting their cleanings on time and thinking their mouths were healthy. They were never told they had the beginnings of periodontal disease. You need to make sure you are getting a thorough examination. Catching periodontal disease early means it is easier to take care of the problem and less chance it will lead to tooth loss. It really upsets me when I see a new patient who had gone for cleanings every six months yet showed up with advanced gum disease. The office was just too busy to evaluate and treat the problem. Even worse, the patient was never told. Remember, periodontal disease does not hurt. If it is not evaluated properly, you probably don't even know you have it.

The examination is really the most important part of the visit— and that's the part patients think they should get for free, because that's the way insurance companies have conditioned them. If an examination is not thorough, it doesn't evaluate the gums

The examination is really the most important part of the visit—and that's the part patients think they should get for free.

for periodontal disease, the teeth for cavities, the bite for occlusion, or the soft tissue for infections, abscesses, or oral cancer. Sometimes x-rays aren't even taken.

I got a mailing at my house recently from a local dentist. On the mailing it said, "Free examination. Free cleaning. Free x-rays." I am sure he got some patients from this, but what do you get for free? What type of practice does this doctor have where he needs to give things away for free to get new patients. All I am saying is be aware. Don't close your eyes to the obvious. You get what you pay for—and if you pay nothing, you probably are not getting what you need.

CAN YOU TRUST YOUR DENTIST?

Because dentists aren't getting the reimbursement needed to cover the cost of a thorough examination, some try to drum up fees in other ways. For example, one of my longtime patients, Roxanne, went to Florida and, while she was there, chipped a tooth. She figured she needed to get it fixed immediately, so she went to a local dentist. He told her she needed seven more crowns in addition to the one for the chipped tooth to make her teeth stronger. Roxanne was very upset. She came back to me and I assured her that she only needed one crown—the one for the broken tooth.

Mary had a similar story. A dentist in another office said she needed a full mouth of crowns as a preventive measure so her teeth wouldn't break. She didn't need any crowns at all! This is just absurd. If you believe this, then everybody should have their teeth crowned. There is nothing better than your own natural teeth. You need to be smart and protect them. When participating in activities like certain sports, it would be wise to wear a custom mouthguard.

Ellen was one of my patients for many years, but economics convinced her to find a dentist who would take her insurance. That was a few years ago. The other dentist made a bridge for her for the top left side of her mouth, but it gave her problems and he never seemed able to fix it. It finally came loose and fell out, so she came back to me and we decided to replace it. So overall, she ended up paying twice for a bridge, because her insurance didn't cover the entire cost of the inferior one. Instead of saving money, she ended up paying more—and that's not even considering the time and aggravation associated with it.

When people go to these offices to save money, very often they're dealing with new dentists who are inexperienced and don't yet understand treatment planning. Often they see a different dentist every time so there's no consistency. These offices are fine for simple procedures like cleanings and simple fillings, but they are not capable of performing complicated dentistry—and they aren't getting paid enough to do it or even present it. They will steer you away from complicated procedures since it's not in their wheelhouse, and recommend only things they feel comfortable doing. This does not mean it is in your best interest. If a dentist does not do implants or know how to restore them, a bridge might be presented instead of a dental implant. This would not be right, but it happens every day.

If a patient's insurance covers a crown a year or a crown every five years, often these operations will tell a patient to get the work done whether they need it or not. Some crowns, if they're done right, literally can last forever. In other cases, if a substandard lab is used or the materials are compromised, that crown might break down sooner rather than later, which means more frequent replacement and shelling out more money out of pocket. Buying cheap really can be more expensive in the long run.

John is another example of a patient who paid a steep price for trying to save a few bucks. He got three root canals done, but they were never restored with crowns, which led him to ultimately lose those three teeth. There are repercussions if procedures aren't done properly.

About 95 percent of dental offices accept some insurance at this point and the numbers are increasing. In addition, there are fewer independent practices as corporations move in and buy out dentists who are finding it more and more difficult to make ends meet. That means patients are losing the intimacy and trust that builds up over the years when they see a single individual.

Also, be weary of the "upsell." As I have mentioned, offices that accept a reduced fee from your insurance company for a procedure need to make up the difference in fee somewhere. All of a sudden you might find that there is a better type of crown available that you can get for an additional fee. You are then paying more money out of pocket than your insurance company has promised you. These "upsells" are very common. Laser gum treatments are normally not a covered procedure. It is true that they can be a benefit in certain circumstances, but not every patient needs them. Many other treatments can be sold to patients at an added expense in order to compensate for the agreement the dentist has made with your insurance company. You might end up paying the same or more than you would be if you went out of your insurance network. An ethical dental practice would not sell you something that you don't need. I am sorry to say, however, that not everybody is ethical. Insurance might cover only a metal crown for a back tooth. If you want porcelain so that it looks like a natural tooth, you'll have to pay more. It's the same when it comes to a bridge—a fixed bridge will cost you more than a removable one. A patient may need gum treatments every three months, but insurance may cover only one a year. Who should be dictating what care you need? Is it your insurance company or your dentist?

It boils down to trust. You need to be able to trust your dentist so that you know you're getting the treatment you need, not just what insurance covers.

ADVANCES IN DENTISTRY

In the recent years, a lot of new materials have come into use. Before, dental amalgams were a mix of mercury and other metals, including silver, tin, and copper—a low-cost mix that can last twenty years. Crowns and bridges had gold. But mercury and gold are giving way to polymer composites and porcelain—even though these materials are much costlier.

The problem is that the cost has forced some dentists to look for cheaper suppliers. The British Dental Industry Association has estimated the black or gray market for dental supplies is a $560 million business, putting both patients and dental staff at risk.[3]

The Dental Trade Alliance, an association of companies that provide dental equipment, supplies, materials, and services to dentists and other oral-care professionals in the United States, Canada, and Mexico, said buying supplies off eBay or Amazon provides no guarantee they have been shipped or stored correctly, let alone whether they've been relabeled or repackaged to conceal an expiration date. More than twelve thousand pieces of illegal dental equipment were seized in the United Kingdom alone during a six-month period in 2014.[4]

In corporate offices, a clerk may be making purchasing decisions based on spending parameters handed down from the executive level. That person doesn't work with the materials and may be unaware they are below standard. It may take a long time before the situation is corrected.

But of course, dentistry still is changing, with researchers working on ways to fill cavities with a biocompatible material that gets teeth to repair themselves. Others are researching ways to arrest decay once it has started, and still others are working on ways of wiping out the acid-producing bacteria that cause decay in the first place.[5]

The point is, all of this costs money.

Among the advantages of going to an individually owned office is that the dentist likely has been there for years. That means continuity of care—something that's missing in corporately owned

3   "The Proliferation of Fake Dental Materials," The London Lingual Orthodontic Clinic, March 24, 2015, https://www.londonlingualbraces.com/for-professionals/the-proliferation-of-fake-dental-materials/

4   Ibid.

5   Marc S. Reisch, "New Materials Take a Bite Out of Tooth Decay," Chemical and Engineering News 94, no. 31 (August 2016): 16–19, https://cen.acs.org/articles/94/i31/New-materials-take-bite-tooth.html

offices because of the turnover of personnel. I can track a patient's periodontal disease. I also know what procedures already have been done and can assess their efficacy. Some people's disease progresses slowly. Others aren't that lucky. The continuity helps me determine what a patient might need. It's just like going to a medical doctor: You want to see the same person all the time—because that person is familiar with your needs.

> Among the advantages of going to an individually owned office is that the dentist likely has been there for years. That means continuity of care—something that's missing in corporately owned offices because of the turnover of personnel.

THE YOUNGER GENERATION

Oral hygiene is an even worse problem among millennials than for previous generations. A recent study commissioned by Hello Products indicated that 30 percent of young adults brush their teeth only once a day, yet half are afraid of losing their teeth due to their poor habits. Nearly a quarter of the two thousand people surveyed said they don't go to the dentist because they don't like the way products taste, and 62 percent said they're just plain scared, so they don't go at all.[6]

These young adults have had to deal with a difficult economy as well as a tough time finding jobs, so maybe they are reluctant to shell out the money for quality care. The internet also is a contributing factor. They look up symptoms online and self-diagnose, thinking

---

6   Sam Paul, "Millennials Are Terrible at Keeping Their Teeth Clean," New York Post, February 23, 2018, https://nypost.com/2018/02/23/millennials-are-terrible-at-keeping-their-teeth-clean/

if it doesn't hurt, they need not go to the dentist. They're also more likely to consume beverages that are bad for their teeth and may not understand the link between a healthy mouth and overall health.

A survey by the ADA indicated that 40 percent of millennials would be happy if they could get their dental care at a CVS, Walgreens, or Target store.[7] I'm a firm believer that we'll eventually see the worst teeth in a half century, because the quality of care is being driven by price. Standards are dropping just as fees are. Quality dentistry cannot be done at the bargain-basement prices insurance is willing to pay. Millennials may want insurance to pay for everything, but keep in mind, the insurance companies don't care about you.

In choosing a dentist, there are a number of things you should take into consideration. As I said earlier, look around the office to make sure the carpet isn't threadbare, and the wallpaper isn't peeling. Then there's the dentist himself. Check out the certificates on the wall. Is there more than just a diploma from dental school? Ask if the dentist takes continuing-education classes regularly. Is the equipment in the office up-to-date, or is the dentist about to retire and making do with the same equipment he has used for decades? Does the dentist explain what is involved in a procedure before doing it? Is the staff personable and helpful?

Dentists are artists. It takes years to get really good. Dental work involves sculpting, visualizing in three dimensions, and medical expertise. That's what separates the good dentists from the not-so-good ones. How many implants has a dentist done—ten or a thousand?

A dentist needs to earn your trust. We're here to educate our patients. We discuss the different ways of fixing something. Unlike

---

7   "Are Millennials Interested in Receiving Dental Care in a Retail Setting?" American Dental Association, Health Policy Institute, June 2016, https://www.ada.org/~/media/ADA/Science%20and%20Research/HPI/Files/HPIgraphic_0716_2.pdf?la=en.

internal medicine where the solution for appendicitis is removing the appendix, in dentistry there may be several approaches. Ask what the various approaches are, and by all means, get a second opinion if you've got reservations. Just like buying a car: Do you take the first vehicle you see on the lot, or do you shop around? Your teeth are an even more important investment. If you're shopping for price, remember: You get what you pay for. There's a direct correlation between fees and what a given dentist can offer.

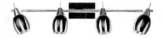

Chapter 4

COMPUTERS, SCANNERS, AND NEW MATERIALS AND TECHNIQUES

D
o you wait anxiously for the next iPhone to come out? What about cars? Do you trade in every few years because you want one with all the new bells and whistles? If that's the case, why should you settle for a dentist who hasn't updated his equipment in years?

Think about it. The most dramatic advances in dentistry have been made in the last twenty-five years, with the last five years seeing an explosion in new materials and techniques. Doesn't your mouth deserve the benefit of all this advancement?

My goal is to make your natural teeth last as long as possible. It doesn't mean they will last forever, but I want to get as close to that as possible. When I fix a tooth, the fix may not last forever, either. There's no material stronger than the teeth with which you were born. I'm very conservative. We start with a small filling. Then we may go to a bigger filling, followed by an onlay, crown, root canal, and implant. We don't want to jump from a small filling to a crown. There are a lot of dentists, however, who put crowns on teeth when people don't need them, shortening the lifespan of the tooth.

I'm not here to convince you of anything. Rather, I'm here to educate you about what is available. And remember, *available* doesn't mean *cheap*. There's a price to be paid for all this technology. Just look at your phone and your car. I'll bet when you bring your car in for service, it gets plugged into a diagnostic computer to determine if there is a problem. We're not at the point where we can plug humans in—but think about the tricorder used on *Star Trek*. In essence, it's a handheld scanner. Someday, the use of a gadget like that might become the norm.

> And remember, *available* doesn't mean *cheap.*

WHAT IS DENTISTRY?

Dentistry is a branch of medicine. As I mentioned earlier, medical and dental students share the same course of study for the first two years of their medical/dental education. Go into a hospital and you'll see everything is computerized. Doctors and nurses have mobile terminals and displays. Scanners and computers monitor blood pressure, breathing, heart rate, oxygen intake, and myriad other things.

So, why accept a dentist who has ignored such advancements? New techniques in dentistry are just as important as the advances made in other branches of medicine. Technology allows us to do things faster, better, and more easily for the patient. It enhances our diagnostic ability and our ability to make patients comfortable.

Granted, not all dental procedures are medical.[8] An overbite is a dental condition and it is treated solely by your dentist, not your

---

8   Christine Taxin, "What Makes It Medical? A Basic Guide to Medical vs. Dental Procedures," *Dentistry IQ*, June 22, 2016, http://www.dentistryiq.com/articles/2016/06/what-makes-it-medical-a-basic-guide-to-medical-vs-dental-procedures.html.

MD. On the other hand, an abscessed tooth is a medical condition. Diabetes is a medical condition that has implications for dental health, especially gum disease.[9] Your dentist needs to be able to recognize and deal with all of it.

Just like your internist, your dentist is a diagnostician. Your internist will run numerous tests and scans to determine what's ailing you. Shouldn't your dentist be able to do the same in determining the best course of treatment for your mouth? After all, you want your teeth to last as long as possible.

Computers, scanners, and other equipment are expensive. It amazes me when a patient comes in for the first time and says he or she never has seen anything like it before. When you go to the dentist, you should expect the same or better service than you get from a mechanic. Computers are integral to the process from the initial consultation to the discussion of procedures to the end of the visit when we go over billing and payments. They're used in every single aspect of the process.

At Advanced DDS, before you even walk into our office, we will e-mail forms to be filled out. You can do them at your leisure and not waste time during your appointment, and we'll still get everything we need. Once you arrive, your picture is taken so we can identify our patients on sight. Then we sit down at a terminal with you and review the forms.

After your information has been reviewed, you have a one-on-one interview with one of our doctors to go over what is needed. You need an x-ray? No problem. Did you know digital x-ray machines

---

9   "Diabetes and Oral Health Problems," American Diabetes Association, Living with Diabetes, September 18, 2012, last modified, May 9, 2018, http://www.diabetes.org/living-with-diabetes/treatment-and-care/oral-health-and-hygiene/diabetes-and-oral-health.html

deliver 80 percent less radiation than standard x-ray equipment?[10] Traditional x-rays use light-sensitive film and need 0.005 millisievert (how radiation is measured) for four bitewings (x-rays of the crowns of the upper and lower teeth)—less than one day's worth of natural background radiation or about the same amount of radiation you get from a two-hour plane ride. Then the film needs to be developed before the dentist can see what's going on. Switch to digital x-rays, which use sensors and transmit the pictures directly to a computer, and the amount of radiation exposure is even more miniscule. I've been doing digital x-rays for decades, one of the first dentists in New York state to do so. Some offices still aren't using them.

Another piece of digital equipment is the intraoral camera, which also has been around for a while. It allows the patient to see what the dentist sees and enables the patient to participate in the decision-making. It allows us to explain our recommendations more fully, enabling the patient to understand why a particular procedure is necessary.

Then there's the DIAGNOdent, a laser that can detect decay. In the old days, a dentist might have looked at a stain on a tooth and not been sure whether that stain represented decay. There were two choices: Watch the tooth for a while to see if decay becomes apparent or drill and fill, just in case. The DIAGNOdent takes the guesswork out of the process. It prevents the dentist from doing something unnecessary yet allows a problem to be treated very early when it is small.

CONE BEAM COMPUTED TOMOGRAPHY SCANNERS (CT OR CAT SCANNERS)

What really has revolutionized dental treatment is the cone beam computed tomography scanner—more commonly known as CBCT.

---

10 X-ray Risk Calculator, *X-ray Risk.com*, last modified January 28, 2018, http://www.x-rayrisk.com/faq.php.

An x-ray produces a two-dimensional picture, good enough for detecting decay and fractures but provides no depth. A CBCT scan, on the other hand, combines the power of x-rays and computers to produce a 360 degree, cross-sectional view in just thirty seconds. It really lets us see what's going on in the jaw, so we can accurately determine how much bone there is for implants and where the important structures like nerve canals are. In short, it allows us to work more accurately and safely. If I know exactly where a nerve is, it's much less likely there will be a problem.

At first, we used the CBCT scanners just for implants, and they became the standard of care in the implant field. You really shouldn't have an implant surgically placed without having a CBCT scan done first. Just because your dentist hasn't invested in this technology doesn't mean you don't need it. After using them for a while, I realized they'd be invaluable for root canals and oral surgery for removing wisdom teeth. You don't need a CBCT scanner for every procedure, but when you do need it, it makes all the difference.

Let me explain how CBCT scanners make doing implants easier. I've been doing implants for decades. When I started, we just had x-rays. The pictures were a bit distorted, and we had to draw on them to show where the implant would go. We essentially were guessing, since we had only height, not width. Using the CBCT scans, we can do all the planning on a computer. We can determine the exact size and angle, and create a guide that can be used to place the implant in the exact position necessary. Think of it as a CAD program similar to what engineers use in building bridges and other structures. We're making a 3-D image and translating it into the mouth. We know exactly where to drill holes. The process is faster, more accurate, and more successful. Spending time planning the implant surgery on a computer reduces the surgical time significantly. The visit is shorter and the implants are placed in the optimal restorative position.

Now let's turn to root canals. Just like you need to snake your drains, sometimes the canals in the teeth need to be cleared of debris and infection. A standard x-ray allows the dentist to see what the tooth looks like, but not what's going on inside. The goal is to seal the tooth off so no more bacteria can enter, thus putting off the time when an implant will be necessary. Sometimes the canals or pipes in the tooth are very small and difficult to find. If a dentist can't find the canal, the tooth cannot be sealed properly. If the infection returns, the root canal has failed, and the patient may wind up losing the tooth. In the past, it could take hours to discover where these canals were hiding. The CBCT scan cuts what used to be an hour-long process to just a few minutes.

The CBCT generates pictures of the soft tissue and nerve paths as well as the bone (x-rays show only the bone). A patient should remove jewelry, glasses, dentures, and hairpins before a scan, since those objects may affect the picture. Some hearing aids and piercings also may need to be removed. These machines are smaller and less expensive than a conventional CT scanner but produce similar images. The cone beam CT scanner provides full diagnostic information and uses less radiation than a conventional CT.

Advanced DDS has a "green" CBCT scanner. It's a low-radiation unit that would expose the patient to about the same amount of radiation as a flight from New York to Los Angeles. In other words, it's not something about which you need to worry.

I've had patients tell me they didn't want any type of x-ray. I've had parents tell me not to x-ray their children's teeth. These parents also refuse to use fluoride toothpaste or allow their children to drink fluoridated water. A year later, the kids come in for root canals. There's always a cost/benefit risk. In the case of digital x-rays and CBCT scans, the benefits far outweigh the risks. Refusing x-rays and CBCT scans forces the dentist to work with eyes closed. It's like the difference between a 15-watt bulb and a 300-watt bulb. I'd rather turn down the work than have a patient dictate to me that I have to work in the dark.

HOW WE FIT A CROWN

Digital impressions have made the whole process of fitting crowns much easier. In the old days, the dentist would fill a tray with goop, shove it into your mouth, and then press hard to make sure there was an adequate impression of the shape of the tooth. Then you would sit there for a while to let the material harden, after which the dentist would remove the tray. There was a bit of wiggling involved. Sometimes the impression would be damaged in the process. A mold was cast and sent out to a lab for processing—a process that could take two weeks or more—and a temporary crown was fitted into the mouth. While you were waiting for the permanent crown, the temporary one might fall out, which meant a trip back to the dentist to have it put back.

Digital impressions and in-office milling technology reduce that two-week or more wait to ninety minutes. Digital impressions and CAD/CAM systems make the process more comfortable, faster, and better than in the past.

Digital scanners allow us to design the restoration right on the computer. We then push a button. Our milling machine takes a block of ceramic and mills out the restoration in just fifteen minutes. I've done thousands of these. The patient gets the crown in one visit, and the crown fits better. Crowns are now made to look more like natural teeth—no more gold or other metal—and they're stronger, function better, and last longer than metal or soft porcelain.

NEWER, STRONGER, BETTER

Recently, a lot of new materials have been introduced, not just for crowns but for fillings as well. Those old silver fillings actually weaken teeth. You know how a sidewalk cracks because of water expanding and contracting? The same thing happens with silver fillings in teeth. What we did in the old days was just drill holes and fill them in. These new materials actually bond with the tooth, reinforcing and holding it together, not just plugging the hole. It's changing the way dentistry is done.

You may have heard that silver amalgams contain mercury. Mercury is a poisonous chemical, but there really isn't enough mercury in a filling to make it dangerous. Holistic dentists want to take out and replace every silver filling. They'll make a lot of money doing that, but it really isn't necessary.

I haven't placed a sliver filling in fifteen years, but not because of the mercury. I haven't placed a silver filling because they cause hairline fractures in teeth. The new porcelain restorations are designed not to do that. Zirconium-oxide ceramics closely resemble the natural tooth, making them ideal for crowns and bridges. Lithium disilicate glass ceramic is used for numerous purposes and can be combined with zirconium-oxide for bridges on rear teeth. In short, these materials are stronger and much more biocompatible; they're great ways to fill in the missing part of a tooth.

More and more new materials are coming on the market. They keep teeth stronger and last longer than materials used in the past. New bonding materials help ceramics stay in place.

For bigger jobs involving multiple teeth, we use digital printers to make models. These models are saved in our database and can be used again if a model is broken. I can print a new model anytime. We also use these printers for night guards for people who grind their teeth and for the surgical guides used for implants. Technically, I can see someone in the morning and do the guided surgery that afternoon. We're now doing digital dentures as well. Labs still mill out the dentures, but we can print try-in steps in the office to save time. We can't yet print permanent crowns, but we can print temporary ones if a case is too complex to resolve in one appointment.

Dentures are notorious for discomfort. The old joke is that we tell the patient we're charging for the top denture but providing the bottom denture for free. There's always more trouble with the bottom denture, because there's less bone with which to work and the ridge is flatter. When a patient complains that the bottom denture is ill-fitting, we then can say, "What do you expect for free?" But kidding aside, we can produce a much more comfortable, better-fitting denture merging digital technology and implant dentistry.

COMPUTER-AIDED ANESTHESIA

Computers also have revolutionized the way we administer anesthesia. STA—single tooth anesthesia—allows a dentist to numb a single tooth rather than the whole mouth. Computer-controlled systems first were introduced in 1997, enabling the dentist to use less pressure for injections and to better calibrate the amount of anesthetic being delivered. Some patients are very hard to anesthetize, and millennials are afraid dental work will hurt. This is a better way of getting them comfortable.

Sarah was one of those patients who never seemed to get numb—the anesthetic would not work on her, and the procedures would hurt. She'd always had a bad experience at the dentist. Rather than sending her home, we used STA "single tooth, computerized anesthesia" on her. She was numb and comfortable in thirty seconds.

So, now you know about all the bells and whistles. What really holds this together is the way the components are sequenced. If I'm doing a full-mouth restoration, this cuts down the number of necessary visits by at least half. The restorations are more accurate, better fitting, more comfortable, and better looking. Most dentists are not trained in digital dentistry. Dental school does not teach these new techniques. They are too busy teaching the basics. This is a problem when I look to add more dentist to my practice. Each time a new dentist is added to Advanced DDS, they are trained in digital dentistry. This has become a game changer for both the dentist and my patients.

Toby came in for a six-hour sedation appointment. He needed three root canals, three crowns, and some fillings. Without digital dentistry, it would have taken three to five visits. If each tooth had been done individually by conventional means, it might have meant nine or ten visits. Instead, it was one and done.

All this technology is expensive—$500,000 to $1 million—and many dentists just don't want to invest, especially older dentists who are eying retirement. Patients need to decide what type of dentistry they want done. Is mediocre good enough or do you want the best?

And you need to ask questions. I've had new patients come in and say their dentists never told them about any of this, and they wish they had known. Yes, it's expensive but there are benefits. The time savings alone may make it worth it.

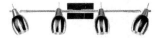

Chapter 5

HOW SEDATION DENTISTRY CAN BENEFIT YOU

You walk into the doctor's or dentist's office. Your blood pressure spikes. Your heart pounds. Along with that comes the sweats. Panic sets in. It's fight or flight.

Why is that? You haven't been to the dentist in years, but every time you think about getting your teeth checked, you feel a sense of dread.

Guess what? You're not alone. It's called white coat hypertension, and an estimated 30 million to 40 million people have that reaction at the dentist's. I see terrified patients every day who only have managed to overcome their fears because the pain in their mouths became too great or they were tired of not being able to smile without embarrassment or were having trouble eating. The first step toward a healthy mouth was taken when they picked up the phone and called or texted for an appointment. (In fact, we have found that texting or e-mailing is less anxiety-inducing when it comes to taking that first step than a direct phone conversation.) Once the overture is made, we can begin the process of retraining the brain to help reduce fears that have built up over a lifetime.

As of this writing, I have been in practice for more than thirty-five years and have gained great insight into the phobic dental patient. Nearly everyone who is afraid of going to the dentist has a story to tell: Something sparked the fear and avoidance behavior. I've heard them all:

- My dentist never used novocaine when I was a kid.

- My dentist said raise your hand if it hurts and I'll stop (but he didn't).

- My dentist drilled into a nerve.

- My dentist pulled a tooth before the novocaine took effect.

- My dentist cut my tongue with the drill.

- My dentist couldn't get me numb but started the work anyway.

- My dentist kept sticking me with needles, but I still felt everything.

- My dentist made me choke while taking molds of my teeth.

- My dentist had bad breath.

There's more, but you get the idea. Now, let's talk about it.

Other than a pinch from the administration of local anesthetic, nothing ever should hurt. I mean it! Pain control has improved greatly over the years. In fact, we don't use novocaine anymore (even though everybody still refers to whatever anesthetic is used as novocaine) because newer agents work faster and are more effective than the old standby.

In the time I've been practicing, I've never used novocaine. The term is used just like Kleenex and Thermos—brand names that people use generically. When was the last time you asked for a tissue instead of a Kleenex, even when the box read Scotties or Puffs or was emblazoned with a store brand? Same thing with insulated bottles. We refer to one as a Thermos.

Before 1905, when Procaine was developed, cocaine was used as a local anesthetic.[11] It was injected into the lower jaw to dull the pain of tooth extraction beginning in the 1880s. Among the drawbacks was that dentists developed a taste for the euphoria-inducing substance, as well, and many died. Procaine had all the desired pain-numbing effects of cocaine but none of its addictive potential. One company introduced the brand name Novocain, which later became novocaine. Lidocaine was discovered in 1946 and now is the most common local anesthetic in dentistry. Numbness lasts thirty minutes to three hours. There is also articaine, which was first synthesized in 1969 and first became popular in Europe. It begins wearing off within two hours. Both lidocaine and articaine are extremely effective.

WHAT MAKES PEOPLE FEARFUL?

There are reasons why people react in certain ways. Their brains have been trained to associate words or actions with specific behaviors. The word dentist may create anxiety because of a bad experience—or more than one. If, however, that bad experience can be replaced with good ones, we can change the way people think about the dentist. Over time, their brains will learn to react positively rather than negatively, because the fear factor has been reduced or even eliminated.

I've seen evidence of this many times. Take Lindsey, for example. She was a new patient who needed a replacement filling because the old restoration had deteriorated (remember, fillings and other restoratives don't last forever). It was a simple procedure, something we do

---

11   Nicholas Calcaterra, "Cocaine and Dentistry," *Directions in Dentistry*, April 23, 2013, http://directionsindentistry.net/cocaine-dentistry-local-anesthetic/.

every day. Well, simple for me, anyway. For Lindsey, it was a different story. She was afraid of the needle with the anesthetic. She was afraid of the drill and its high-pitched whine. She didn't like the stuffing in her mouth to soak up the saliva and keep the soft tissue away from the work site. But she was a trooper and let me proceed. I replaced the filling without incident. Afterward, she said it was the best filling she had ever had. What she really was saying was that it was the best dental experience she had ever had—she hadn't felt a thing.

What surprised me was that it was just a filling. I've been doing those the same way, day in and day out, for years. Apparently, some other dentists don't take the time or have the ability to make sure their patients are comfortable. I try to treat the whole patient, not just the teeth. I want to make sure a patient feels good about what is being done. Showing sympathy and compassion and respecting a patient's fears, often is enough to reduce the anxiety. For cases where that's not enough, there's always sedation.

CHOOSING THE RIGHT SEDATION

Over time, sedation dentistry has evolved. Oral surgeons always have provided sedation. They receive their sedation training as they receive their surgical training, becoming adept at everything from conscious sedation to general anesthesia. Unlike oral surgeons, general dentists usually don't get sedation training during their studies. It's something that really should be added to the curriculum.

As a result, general dentists have tried different methods of soothing anxious patients. When I was a child, I remember my dad experimenting with white noise and hypnosis as soothing agents. Dad always was interested in keeping his patients comfortable. But the truth is, neither of these really was effective and many people still avoided going in for dental work.

The idea of using white noise first was introduced in 1959, but studies on its effectiveness have been mixed.[12] The idea is to distract the patient, causing sensory confusion to suppress pain. It's about as effective as breathing exercises when you have cramps. Dad didn't stick with it for very long.

Hypnosis was a hot topic for several years as a means of keeping fearful patients comfortable, and though it may help a patient relax and relieve some anxiety, it does little to alleviate pain.[13] But hypnosis is not magic, and the more anxious a patient is, the less likely a trance will be induced.[14]

Nitrous oxide, also known as laughing gas, has been in use for decades. It's a very common, sweet-smelling inhaled anesthetic that reduces anxiety and pain sensitivity. For the patient who is only mildly anxious, nitrous oxide might be enough to take the edge off and allow a procedure to be accomplished in a comfortable, non-stressful way. One of the advantages of nitrous oxide is that it has no aftereffects. Patients can eat before an appointment and can drive themselves home, since the gas is eliminated swiftly by the body. A doctor doesn't need any kind of special training to use this mild form of sedation. For most patients, even children, it is extremely safe and effective. The mildly apprehensive patient also can be treated effectively with a combination of a good local anesthetic and nitrous oxide.

But what about the patient whose blood pressure goes up, accompanied by cold sweats and a pounding heart? The moderately

12 Laura A. Mitchell et al., "A Survey Investigation of the Effects of Music Listening on Chronic Pain," *Psychology of Music* 35, no. 1 (January 2007), https://doi.org/10.1177/0305735607068887

13 Gow, Mike, "Hypnosis," *DentalFearCentral.org*, accessed 2018, https://www.dentalfearcentral.org/help/psychology/dental-hypnosis/.

14 Facco E., G. Zanette, and E. Casiglia, "The Role of Hypnotherapy in Dentistry", *SAAD Digest* 30, (January 2014): 3–6, https://www.ncbi.nlm.nih.gov/pubmed/24624516.

to severely apprehensive patient needs more than a local anesthetic and/or nitrous oxide. That's where sedation dentistry comes in. There currently are two forms of sedation: oral and IV. Oral sedation involves swallowing a pill, and in IV sedation, the sedative is injected directly into the bloodstream.

Oral sedation became popular around 1999 when Drs. Anthony Feck and Michael Silverman partnered to establish DOCS Education, an organization established to teach dentists how to administer oral sedation, which generally involves benzodiazepines to reduce anxiety and provide sedative effects, amnesia, muscle relaxation, and anti-convulsive effects. DOCS Education provided training throughout the United States, enabling many dentists to provide safe and effective oral sedation for patients who needed it. Now, you'll find most dentists provide the service. Dentists can take a two-day course from DOCS or other providers to learn to administer oral sedatives. To determine whether your dentist is certified for oral sedation, check the government webpage.

The advantage of oral sedation is simple. Just swallow a pill. Most dentists are not trained in IV sedation, and there are patients who don't want needles in their arms. But those are the only advantages. The list of drawbacks is much lengthier.

Oral sedation is difficult to control. Because it goes through the digestive system, the rate of absorption into the bloodstream is unpredictable. It also takes a while, maybe an hour or more to take effect. If not enough medication is administered the first time, another dose is given and more waiting is involved. If too much is administered, it could take hours to wear off, and the patient will feel drowsy and sedated for the rest of the day. That means a short procedure could turn into a daylong affair, during which the patient needs to be monitored fully—blood pressure, pulse, oxygen concentration, breathing, heart. So don't be surprised if you are wired up to equipment before the procedure.

Oral sedation is safe, but everything must be done properly. Another disadvantage to oral sedation is that it cannot be reversed rapidly or easily if too much was administered. Because there's no direct route into the bloodstream, medication used to reverse the drugs needs to be administered in other ways. Reversal generally is not needed, but without an intravenous route, it's also not as effective when it is needed. The reversal drug flumazenil is administered through submucosal or sublingual injections "under the tongue" but it can take as long as three minutes to work. Patients who use benzodiazepines to control seizures may suffer a seizure if flumazenil is used.

This takes us to IV sedation, something very few general dentists—or even specialists other than oral surgeons—offer. The training is more rigorous than other forms of sedation and most dentists are not interested in adding this to their repertoire. To them it's not worth the time or effort it would take to get proficient. They generally never were trained in putting in an IV or in handling emergency situations. Of the thousands of dentists on Long Island, New York, only a few offer IV sedation—and the figures aren't much different in the rest of the country.

I saw the need for sedation dentistry in my practice years ago. Many patients who were getting implants wanted to be "put out" for the procedures. That meant bringing in an anesthesiologist, which added to the expense. When the DOCS certification became available, I was one of the first dentists to go through the training in New York state. I offered it for a year or two for implant surgery, and it worked pretty well. But I wanted something more effective. That's when I got my certification for IV sedation from Montefiore Medical Center in the Bronx, eliminating the need to hire an anesthesiologist and thus reducing the cost to my patients.

IV sedation has many advantages. First, it acts quickly. Usually, we can start a procedure within a few minutes of starting a drip. Compare that to the hour it takes for oral sedation to work. The dosage can be controlled easily, eliminating the chances of giving too much or too little. The medication is short-acting, enabling patients to walk out of the office on their own power rather than needing wheelchairs.

The same equipment needed to monitor patients for oral sedation is needed in IV sedation. We use an electrocardiogram to monitor the heart; there's also a pulse monitor, blood pressure monitor, blood-oxygen monitor, and capnography to monitor breathing.

It didn't take me long to realize IV sedation had more applications than just for implants. After a year or two, I opened my sedation practice to any form of dentistry. Patients who in the past preferred having a tooth pulled to undergoing a root canal finally had an alternative. If they could be sedated for an extraction, why not sedate them for a procedure that would save the tooth? I even provide sedation for cleanings. If it makes patients more likely to take care of their teeth, why not?

So which form of sedation is best for you or someone you know who avoids going to the dentist? The decision should be based on the procedure involved and determined by the patient together with the dentist. You need to trust your provider to help you figure out what you need.

Many people come into Advanced DDS after seeing our television commercial on fearful patients and sedation dentistry. We advertise for a reason. Most fearful patients think they are unique. They're not. Approximately 10 percent of the population fears going to the dentist and does not know the work can be done comfortably in a relaxed atmosphere. They see my commercial and they come in.

I would say about half of these patients just want a place that understands their fears. Some people just need to see a friendly, caring face. Those a little more apprehensive may just need a touch of nitrous oxide. Others need to be sedated before I can even look at their teeth.

I always tell my patients I won't hurt them: hurting them benefits no one. If I hurt them, they won't be back, so we'd both lose. I prefer we both win. We get happy patients, and they get their dentistry done in a manner they never thought possible.

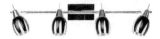

Chapter 6

A HEALTHY MOUTH CONTRIBUTES TO A HEALTHY BODY

At Advanced DDS, we're dedicated to providing full-service, family dentistry to keep not only our patients' mouths healthy but the rest of their bodies as well. Some people avoid the dentist until the pain in their mouths becomes unbearable. At that point, oral neglect may have led to other serious health problems.

Your regular checkup can keep some problems at bay or uncover underlying health conditions that have not yet become apparent to your internist. The pain in your mouth may mean there's an infection that can spread elsewhere. Remember, we can take away your pain painlessly.

What am I talking about when I say oral health? Teeth aren't the only structures in the oral cavity. Decayed or broken teeth contribute to pain and poor function, and can lead to other complications. It's important to understand, however, there are other structures in the mouth that need attention, including the gums, bone, soft tissue, and tongue.

The effects of many diseases, conditions, and habits also manifest in the mouth: diabetes, cardiovascular disease, sleep apnea, osteoporosis, digestion, respiratory infections, TMJ (temporomandibular joint) pain and function, and pregnancy. Smoking, chewing tobacco, and consuming beverages (both alcoholic and nonalcoholic) can also cause problems in the mouth.

Let's examine each of these.

TEETH

We all know what teeth are. These solid structures with nerves and a blood supply in the center form in the gums. Baby teeth erupt during infancy, permanent teeth during childhood, and wisdom teeth during adolescence or early adulthood. Front teeth are for cutting and back teeth are for chewing. Over time, through use and environmental factors, teeth become worn, broken, and/or decayed. "So what?" you might say. My parents lost their teeth; I probably will too.

If you lose your teeth, then what? We can replace your teeth, gums, and lost bone with plastic. We call these dentures. People expect these plastic structures to work the same way their natural teeth once did, but in reality, there is no way you can expect a piece of plastic to function as well as the teeth with which you were born. So, knock down your expectation level. There's nothing better than your natural teeth, even if you have crowns, veneers, or even implants. In an ideal world, your teeth would last a lifetime, but this doesn't always happen. Whether through wear, accidents, or decay, teeth can be lost. We're still years away from being able to regenerate teeth. In the meantime, it's important that they be replaced as they are lost. Let's talk about why.

If spaces are left in our mouths by missing teeth, it's not a matter of just eating on the other side. The remaining teeth shift, becoming crooked and cocked at odd angles. This contributes to gum disease and bone loss and can lead to the loss of even more teeth. If enough teeth are missing, it's hard to eat. Your digestion is affected. So is your overall health.

Your digestive system starts in your mouth. The teeth grind and mash the food, so saliva can start breaking it down and lubricating the food before it's swallowed. Losing teeth is the first step in making the digestive system less effective. If you can't chew adequately, you'll need to swallow larger pieces, which is difficult. That can lead to weight loss, which in turn can lead to many other health problems. Not chewing food adequately also can cause stomach upset and acid reflux.

Sometimes teeth can decay without pain. I had a patient whose teeth were broken to the gum line, yet he never experienced any discomfort. Without pain, there was no incentive to undergo treatment. Often on examination, I find multiple infections in the jaw around broken teeth. Such infections may remain local, but sometimes they spread to other parts of the mouth and up into the sinuses. Sometimes they spread to the throat and interfere with breathing. In rare cases, they can work their way to the brain or heart and cause death.

Joe came in with a failing root canal. It had been failing for a while. The site was an upper tooth next to his sinus cavity. He'd had sinus problems on that side of his face for many years but had not received proper treatment. After the infected tooth was removed, his sinus problems cleared up almost immediately. He could not believe he had lived with the discomfort for so long when the problem could have been treated easily and swiftly by a dentist.

These infections also can lead to bone loss, a major concern for women on medication for osteoporosis. Some of these medications, bisphosphonates (Boniva, Actinal), prevent the jaw bone from regenerating, making jaw infections more probable. Before beginning to take these medications, it's important to get all dental problems resolved. The risk factors are small, but if a person on bisphosphonates has an infection or needs dental surgery like an extraction, osteone-crosis of the jaw could develop, actually killing the jaw bone. This is a debilitating disease that's very difficult to cure. If you are taking one of these medications or plan to start, talk to your doctor about the risks and let your dentist know.

SOFT TISSUE

The soft tissue that lines the cheeks, floor of the mouth, tongue, and throat also can become infected or even cancerous. Squamous cell carcinoma is an oral cancer that can be lethal. Your dentist should do an oral cancer screening at least once a year as part of the examination. There also are advanced screenings that can be performed that work better than a visual examination. These advanced screenings involve different types of light that show changes to the soft tissue before such changes are obvious to the naked eye in normal lighting. Ask your dentist if he or she has this type of equipment. Catching precancerous lesions early can save your life.

And what are the major causes of oral cancer? You guessed it: smoking and chewing tobacco. I'm not going to lecture you about it. I just have one thing to say: STOP. We all know smoking causes lung cancer. The link has been apparent for decades. But, think about where the smoke first hits. The mouth, then the throat. Smoke is an irritant and toxin. The heat from the smoke also works as an irritant. Any tissues can be affected. How do you know if there's a problem? Look for red and white areas in the mouth that don't look as if they belong, ulcers and sores that don't go away, sores that are present but don't hurt (cancer very often does not produce pain), or teeth that become loose for no reason. Anywhere the smoke hits is susceptible.

GUMS

People who are diabetic or borderline diabetic are at a higher risk of gum disease and tooth loss. If diabetes is not controlled and your A1C is higher than seven, you are at risk of implant failure and dental infection. So, what can you do? I'm sure every doctor will tell you to get your A1C below seven—not just to save your teeth, but to save your life. I also ask my patients who have diabetes to come in every three months to get their teeth cleaned for periodontal maintenance. Because a diabetic's risk factors are much higher than people not afflicted with the disease, diabetics need to take even better care of their teeth. Your insurance likely won't cover more than two visits a year. Picking up the other two yourself is a nominal investment. A cleaning is much less expensive than a crown or implant. Diabetics also should remember to schedule their appointments early in the day. If you need sedation, you are not allowed to eat for at least six hours before treatment. Talk to your doctor about how to handle your medication.

Periodontal or gum disease causes the bone around the teeth to melt away. The teeth become loose and eventually can fall out. Gum disease is caused by bacteria and plaque below the gum line, creating inflammation or infection around the gums and surrounding struc-tures. One obvious sign of gum disease is bleeding gums. If you brush your teeth and see blood, chances are you have some gum disease. The early stages are called gingivitis. At this point, the bone supporting the teeth is not yet melting away and treatment is relatively simple. Routine scaling and root planing (removing the plaque and calculus or tartar on the root surfaces) by your hygienist and better home care should take care of it.

Advanced gum disease is another story. If the bone around the teeth has been compromised and teeth are loosening, more advanced treatment would be necessary. This may consist of deep cleanings, laser treatments, or even surgery to try to build back the lost bone.

Even scarier, studies indicate there is a relationship between heart disease and periodontal disease.[15] Bacteria around the teeth and gums can enter the bloodstream and settle in different parts of the body. If it settles around the heart, it could cause a more serious problem than just loose teeth: Namely, endocarditis. The bacteria can latch onto damaged areas inside the heart, generally attacking the valves. People with valve replacements are advised to start taking antibiotics before going to the dentist.

Everyone has bacteria in the mouth, even healthy people. But when advanced periodontal disease is present, the risk of that bacteria spreading elsewhere is much greater. The American Academy of Periodontology reports periodontal disease may increase the risk of respiratory infections like chronic obstructive pulmonary disease and pneumonia.[16] Generally, patients with respiratory diseases had worse periodontal health than those in a control group, the study indicated. Bacteria from the throat or the mouth is inhaled and can be severely debilitating, sometimes leading to death.

Testing for gum disease is simple and should be part of every thorough dental exam. Measurements are taken around the neck of each tooth. These measurements show the degree of bone loss present. During periodontal probing, your doctor should be calling off numbers for each tooth. Between one and three, the tooth is healthy; between four and six, there is moderate disease; numbers greater than

---

15 "Harvard Heart Letter—When an Infection Attacks the Heart," *Harvard Health Publishing*, Harvard Medical School, July 2016, https://www.health.harvard.edu/heart-health/when-an-infection-attacks-the-heart.

16 "Healthy Gums may Lead to Healthy Lungs," *Perio.org*, American Academy of Periodontology, January 18, 2011, https://www.perio.org/consumer/healthy-lungs

six mean advanced periodontal disease is present. This probing should be performed even if insurance doesn't cover it.

SLEEP APNEA

Did you know your dentist can treat sleep apnea? The American Dental Association says dentists are the only health-care providers with the knowledge and expertise to provide oral appliances for sleep apnea therapy.

If you have sleep apnea, you actually stop breathing for much longer than you would if you were holding your breath. The disorder is prevalent and has many long-term repercussions. Most people wake up gasping for breath or gasp for air in their sleep. In the morning, they feel tired, a feeling that lasts throughout the day. Less apparent is how it affects the cardiovascular system by putting tremendous strain on the heart and increasing blood pressure. In fact, it can affect nearly every system in the body.

The Epworth Sleepiness Scale (ESS) is a simple test to help you determine if you should be evaluated for sleep apnea. If you have sleep apnea, it is important to get treatment. Mild to moderate cases can be treated with oral appliances called MRDs—mandibular repositioning devices. These devices keep the lower jaw and tongue forward to keep the airway open. The device is simple and can save your life.

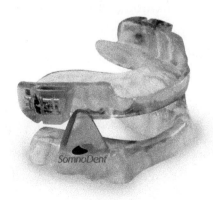

BRUXISM

Teeth grinding, or bruxism, is very common and often the result of stress. Your teeth can age faster than you do if you're a grinder. Craig was just thirty-five years old, but his teeth belonged in the mouth of someone twice his age. They were worn down on all sides and looked like someone took a piece of sandpaper to smooth them out. During the consultation with Craig, we discussed restoring his teeth to their proper function and dealing with the grinding by wearing an appliance at night. At age thirty-five, it is possible to catch this wear early enough before it is irreversible. I have patients that have been grinding their teeth all their lives. By age sixty, their teeth are no longer able to be saved. The bigger problem is how to replace the worn teeth. As the teeth wear down the bone keeps on growing. This makes it very difficult, sometimes even impossible, to rebuild the mouth to its proper function. The best solution is to catch grinding early and listen to your dentist's advice.

Wearing down teeth through grinding can cause many problems. The teeth become shorter and can be more sensitive or even may need root-canal therapy. If the teeth are worn down to the gums, they will need to be replaced with implants. The way the teeth meet will change, causing jaw or TMJ (temporomandibular joint) pain.

Some people have stomach problems; others grind their teeth. It's also likely teeth grinders have other sleep disorders such as snoring and sleep apnea. This destructive habit is tough to stop, largely because it occurs at night when you are sleeping, making it impossible for you to control. Often grinders also clench their jaws during the day, but because it's daytime, they're likely to notice and stop. In other cases, people grind their teeth because their bite is off.

Teeth grinding may be loud enough to wake a partner. It can lead to increased tooth pain or sensitivity, because deeper layers of the tooth become exposed. There can be pain in the jaw, neck, or facial muscles. Sometimes tight muscles won't allow the jaw to open or close completely. The pain can feel like an earache or cause a headache.

Teeth grinding may first manifest in childhood, and people with aggressive personalities are more likely to exhibit the behavior than others. It also can be the result of some medications like antidepressants, or of smoking (another reason to quit), drinking caffeinated beverages or alcohol, or using recreational drugs.

Bruxism also is associated with Parkinson's disease, dementia, gastroesophageal reflux disorder, epilepsy, night terrors, and attention-deficit/hyperactivity disorder.

I recommend wearing an appliance at night called an occlusal or night guard. The device is made of plastic and covers one arch in the mouth, doesn't matter whether it's the lower or upper. Instead of grinding your teeth, you're wearing down the plastic. The other benefit is that the occlusal guard is softer than teeth. People who grind their teeth often wake with jaw pain because all night long the muscles have been working overtime. It's like a nightlong exercise routine. The occlusal guard is designed to allow the muscles to relax and shut down, reducing the grinding and the pain. If your spouse says you grind your teeth while you sleep, talk to your dentist about a custom occlusal guard to prevent your teeth from aging faster than you do.

PREGNANCY

Pregnancy can lead to dental problems in some women, including gum disease and increased risk of tooth decay. Hormones can affect the body's response to plaque. Gums may become puffy and inflamed. Sometimes lesions called pyogenic granulomas form (they're harmless but need to be removed surgically). Also, if the mother-to-be doesn't take in enough calcium, it's her bones, as well as her teeth, that will suffer. Granted, morning sickness, specifically the acid in vomit, may have an impact. But proper home and professional care can keep gum problems and decay at bay.

BEVERAGES

What effect do beverages have on teeth? It's not just sugary drinks that are the problem. Plenty of low-sugar, no-sugar drinks have acid in them, and that acid eats away at the enamel, eroding teeth. Of course, sugary drinks are worse, because bacteria in the mouth turns that sugar into more acid. It's like sucking lemons. The effect is similar to what happens when someone is bulimic. The acid in vomit starts destroying teeth. Then there's the problem of staining. Chromogens in beverages can attach to tooth enamel that has been compromised by the acid.

When it comes to alcoholic beverages, beer is only marginally better than hard liquor or red wine. High alcohol content in a drink can lead to a dry mouth. Saliva is needed to keep teeth moist and to help remove plaque and bacteria from the tooth surfaces. On the bright side, red wine kills oral bacteria, specifically streptococci, which are associated with tooth decay.

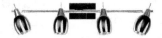

Chapter 7

THE MYTH OF EXPENSIVE DENTISTRY

Think about what happens if you don't take your car in for regular oil changes. The engine components warp and wear out without lubrication. Eventually the engine seizes up and quits. Or the brakes: If you don't replace the pads and make sure you have enough fluid, eventually you won't be able to stop. When your mechanic tells you it's time to have the work done, do you ignore the advice? No. Because you don't want to be without your car, have an accident, or incur the expense of buying a new vehicle.

So, why should you treat your teeth any differently?

Neglect in the long run is more expensive than regular maintenance whether we're talking about cars or mouths. The reason your dentist suggests semiannual visits is because it makes it easier to catch disease early. Early diagnosis generally can prevent the majority of serious dental problems. A basic cleaning is simpler than deep scaling or gum surgery. Small fillings are easier to do and less expensive than root canals, crowns, or implants.

I've heard my patients complain that dental work is expensive. Rather than casting it as a burdensome expense, think of it as an investment in yourself. What are your teeth really worth to you?

I tried a little experiment. I asked some people how much they would want to allow me to extract a healthy tooth—one of their front teeth right where everyone could see. Some people said $10,000; some said $50,000; others said no way, no how. To them just that one tooth was very valuable. But when these same people are told they need a crown, suddenly that's too expensive.

I've heard my patients complain that dental work is expensive. Rather than casting it as a burdensome expense, think of it as an investment in yourself. What are your teeth really worth to you?

Everyone's definition of expensive is different. I think something is too expensive when a person can't afford it. I've had people tell me a treatment is too expensive, but then in the next breath they're bragging about an upcoming trip to Disney for a family of four. Now that's expensive; and after a week, it's gone forever.

What if you come in and I find a small cavity in a molar? It doesn't hurt. In fact, it's just a speck on the x-ray. I tell you it needs to be filled, but you're reluctant to take any action. Time passes, and you just haven't found it convenient to come in for the work. It's six months later and time for your next cleaning. This time, the cavity is a big hole, and you've noticed sensitivity on that side of your mouth from sweet and cold. You've been ignoring it. Now, I say we're past the point where a small filling will take care of it. That filling would have cost a few hundred dollars. But now, you need a root canal and crown on that tooth, which will cost thousands.

It only takes one incident for patients to learn that lesson. The best patients are those who come in regularly every six months, have invested in their mouths, and want to keep that investment healthy.

When cell phones were just beginning to make their appearance, they weren't very sleek or easily portable. They couldn't really do anything besides make and receive phone calls, and even then, you needed to be within a given carrier's range. In fact, a lot of us referred to them as bricks because of their size and weight. But now the devices are a necessity, and Apple, Samsung, and other manufacturers have managed to put a smart phone in nearly everyone's pocket. Even young children carry them. That's pretty remarkable considering the cost of an annual contract; even the cut-rate services are expensive. A family of four could pay upward of $200 a month, $2,400 or more a year, for the ability to use such phones. That same family could visit the dentist twice a year for less. Some people value their phones more than their teeth. A phone can be replaced; your adult teeth can't.

Neglect, I'll say it again, is expensive.

THE REAL COST OF NEGLECT

People complain about having to pay for a cleaning and complain the doctor didn't spend much time with them. I have patients who don't even want the examination, just the cleaning. I have them sign a release explaining there can be an undiagnosed disease present, and without an examination, they're putting themselves at risk. It really surprises me when they insist on cleanings only. The examination is the most important part of the visit. And no, it doesn't take long, but you're paying for the dentist's expertise.

Other people turn down x-rays. They don't want to spend the money or they're afraid of the radiation, which is minimal. I had one family that would not allow me to x-ray the children's teeth for both those reasons. A few years later, the children needed root canal treatment on multiple teeth. Was it really safer and cheaper not to have preventive care and save a few dollars on the x-rays?

There's an old British proverb: penny wise, pound foolish. You cut corners here and there to save money but then wind up spending way more than what was saved when the penury proves to be the wrong choice.

A patient will say, "Okay Doc, just put in another filling. I don't want a crown," or "My kid really doesn't need sealants. Don't do them," or "No x-rays. Maybe next time," or "I don't want to come back in three months for my gums. I'll see you next year for a cleaning," or "I really don't need that back tooth. Just pull it out," or "Don't do a gum treatment. Just clean my teeth," or "Nothing hurts. Let's skip the exam"—or a hundred other things that could wind up being big problems in a year or two or five.

By the time these patients realize there's a problem, the situation is much worse. What could have been handled with a filling now needs a crown or root canal—or maybe the tooth can't be saved at all. These people have become dental invalids. Putting them back together becomes very difficult and expensive.

Taking out the tooth and not putting something in that space presents another group of problems. Teeth begin to shift as soon as space becomes available. The bite changes. Opposing teeth will grow up or down into the space. After a few years, the whole mouth looks different because of that missing tooth. It would have been cheaper and easier to have fixed that tooth or to have replaced it at the time of removal with an implant or bridge than to try to fix the subsequent changes.

Barry recently came in because of swellings and loose teeth. He hadn't seen a dentist in part because of fear and in part because of the expense, but he finally came to his senses. I had to tell him it was too late. Eight teeth needed to be removed because of infection and missing bone. Had he come in for regular visits, that likely would not have been necessary.

Julie was just as bad. Whenever she had a problem, she told the dentist just to extract the tooth. By the time I saw her, half her teeth were missing. She wanted her smile back because she was uncomfortable talking to and having to smile at people at work. It was affecting her self-esteem and quality of life. Restoring her smile meant total dental rehabilitation. I'm sure the cost was much higher than if she had cared for her teeth all along. I've seen this repeatedly.

A QUESTION OF TRUST

As I've said before, you need to go to a dentist you trust. A lot of variables go into deciding whether a tooth is worth saving. You're not going to spend a fortune on one tooth if the rest can't be saved. The mouth has to be evaluated as a whole.

There are two ways of doing dentistry. The first is dealing with one tooth at a time, and that's often what is done in basic dental practices. This is not the best approach. It's possible that all the teeth can be saved, but sometimes, some teeth might need to be sacrificed to save the rest and that takes a more global approach to treatment. If a tooth is broken down to the gum, there might not be enough left to build it back up and it will need to be removed. But it's not all black and white. There are a lot of gray areas. That's where you need to work with your dentist. Will a restoration last five to ten more years? If not, extraction and an implant might be the better route.

To me, dentistry is a sequential process. I can fix almost anything. The question is how long it will last. If we don't do the treatment, you'll lose the tooth. Some patients say if the restoration is not going to last a lifetime, they don't want to spend the money to do the work. Unless the tooth, after being fixed, will last three to five years, an implant is a better choice than a root canal and crown. Before implants were available, a dentist would do anything to save a tooth because there was no alternative. Implants changed the game. They provide more predictability. Why not just cut to the chase and put in an implant?

ADVERTISING AND THE DAMAGE IT CAUSES

The media portrays dentistry as very expensive. It's a hot-button issue in advertising, luring people for free services and cheap dentistry. Insurance companies tell patients they can get their work done more cheaply through their networks. But is that really the answer? Do you put the wrong oil in your car just because it's cheaper? The owner's manual tells you what type to use. Use something different, and you could ruin the engine.

Going cheap is often more expensive down the line. Free rarely really is free. But this is how offices get you into the door. Be wary of free or discounted services.

Corporate dentistry has run commercials in some states telling people dentistry is expensive. They actually say that flat out—boasting that expensive dentists don't work for them. Unbelievable! One of these entities is violating the American Dental Association code that prohibits speaking ill of other dentists. Every dentist runs his or her practice differently based on the population served.

What I'm saying is, think about the type of dentistry you want for yourself. Be informed. You get what you pay for.

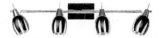

Chapter 8

HOW TO CREATE MAGIC IN YOUR SMILE

A great smile is the best way to make a good first impression. A study by the American Academy of Cosmetic Dentistry indicated 48 percent of adults think a smile is a person's most memorable feature.[17] To be powerful, a smile first must be attractive.

Smile at yourself in the mirror and you can change your attitude for the day. Smiling while answering the phone changes the tone of your voice. I always tell my staff to answer the phone with a smile. We even put mirrors next to the phones to remind them. And Ladies: studies indicate that 70 percent of men think a woman is more attractive when she smiles.[18] Women probably feel the same way about men.

A smile can be a big influence. Smile at a baby and the baby tends to smile back. It makes the baby feel safe and secure. A baby's smile

---

17 "Study Reveals Keys to Memorable First Impressions," AACD Executive Office, American Academy of Cosmetic Dentistry, February 10, 2015, https://www.aacd.com/index.php?module=express&cmd=newsviewpost &id=8005.

18 M. Bendixen, "Evidence of systematic bias in sexual over- and underpercep- tion of naturally occurring events: a direct replication of Haselton (2003) in a more gender-equal culture," *Evol Psychol* 12, no. 5 (November 2014): 1004–21, https://www.ncbi.nlm.nih.gov/pubmed/25402231.

is a delight that often makes the adult feel happy. It's a universal way to communicate with others. It means the same in every language.

Other studies indicate smiling can make you healthier, reducing stress and lowering blood pressure. It stimulates the brain's reward system, making people feel better. Mother Teresa always urged people to meet others with a smile, calling it "the beginning of love." She also said one never knows all the good a simple smile can do. Try walking down a street and smiling at a stranger. Often the stranger will smile right back.

What happens, though, when you are not confident about smiling? Do you cover your mouth with your hand? When photos are taken, do you make sure your teeth are not visible? Do you know someone who does these things? I see patients all the time who do this. One of the first things they say to me is that they want to be able to smile again.

Someone beginning a job search who hasn't been on an interview in years might realize getting a new position would be difficult with missing or broken teeth. Maybe there's a special occasion coming up like a child's wedding, a reunion, or some other event where pictures will be taken. One patient said she decided to do something because her grandchild was making fun of her missing teeth. Whatever it takes. Luckily, we have a number of solutions.

TEETH WHITENING

In recent years, teeth whitening has gained popularity. When I first went into practice, this was a difficult process involving caustic chemicals that could burn the gums. When the dental industry realized there could be big bucks in the procedure, dentists began looking for new and better products. In the 1980s, we discovered that hydrogen peroxide used to treat gum disease had a surprising side effect: It whitened teeth. As a result, gel trays were developed for the purpose. Dentists sold take-home systems fabricated from a patient's dental impressions. Soon big companies got involved. Crest White Strips and imitators came on the market. Brite-Smile whitening became popular—gel would be applied to the teeth and a bright light was used to accelerate the whitening process. Ninety minutes later, a patient's smile was noticeably whiter compared with the weeks that earlier systems took. Whitening toothpastes will whiten teeth over time by a few shades and help keep them whiter. The whitening strips work in a few weeks.

Even more options are available now. The American Academy of Cosmetic Dentistry put the total revenue from teeth whitening in 2015 at $11 billion, with the total expected to continue to climb. Americans paid an average $600 per visit for teeth whitening in a dental office and $35 for at-home kits.

At Advanced DDS, we use Zoom Whitening. This is an in-office system that will whiten teeth as many as seven shades in as little as an hour. The system uses a higher concentration of hydrogen peroxide. There's also a take-home system that is effective and gets quick results; it can be used by itself or as a means of maintenance following in-office whitening.

All these methods work. It just depends how white you want your teeth or how diligent you are about using the take-home systems. Most people prefer immediate gratification and opt for an in-office, hour-long treatment. However, everyone's teeth whiten differently. A lot depends on the color at which we're starting. The darker the teeth, the darker the final result. The process is not 100 percent predictable. And of course, it won't change chipped or crooked teeth. If a tooth needs restoration, it will still need restoration after whitening has been completed.

ORTHODONTICS

Most people have some crooked teeth. Perfectly straight teeth are highly unusual. Conventional orthodontics is done with brackets and wires. Orthodontists get special training in placing these brackets and wires and moving teeth into more aesthetic and functional positions. When we were kids, that was the only option, and most adults were unwilling to go the tinsel-mouth route. But recently, companies such as Invisalign and ClearCorrect have produced clear aligners that move teeth just like brackets and wires, revolutionizing orthodontia and convincing many general dentists to offer the service. It's a very effective method of changing your smile. Please note that gums and teeth need to be in perfect health, however. Moving teeth in an unhealthy mouth can lead to tooth loss.

Some companies are marketing orthodontic systems directly to the public, bypassing the dentist, but this is a mistake that can lead to disaster. Without proper monitoring, moving teeth can cause serious problems—so don't try to be your own orthodontist! I have transformed many smiles with Invisalign and Zoom Whitening. They provide a relatively simple way to create a new you.

PORCELAIN VENEERS

Okay, suppose your teeth are straight but some are chipped, and their shape is off. We can fix that using science to create a pleasing smile. The proportions seen in nature are called the golden ratio or divine proportion: value, 1.618.[19] The golden ratio (a+b/a = a/b) is symbolized by the Greek character φ (phi). The formula has been used in designing buildings such as the Greek Parthenon. In nature, flower

---

19 "Golden Ratio," *MathIsFun.com*, 2015, https://www.mathsisfun.com/numbers/golden-ratio.html

petals are one example of the ratio. You can also find examples of the golden ratio in the face itself: the distance between the eyes and the bottom of the chin. Teeth also follow the golden proportions to measure the shape of the front central incisors compared to the lateral incisors and the eye teeth. A talented dentist with a quality laboratory are able to create a beautiful smile by following these proportions in your smile. This is done with veneers or crowns.

Porcelain veneers can change the size, shape, and color of your teeth to match these golden proportions. The materials used for porcelain veneers have improved markedly in recent years. They are stronger and more aesthetic than ever. The procedure is simple, but the end product, as I said, depends on the quality of the lab and the skill of the dentist. Tooth preparation depends on the condition of the tooth. The veneer is then bonded on. They work really well if shape and color is the only concern. Decayed or broken teeth will need other treatment.

It actually is better to do whitening and straightening than veneers, provided the teeth are in good condition. In the 1980s, we didn't have much choice. The whitening agents were inadequate and straightening was something most people thought was just for teenagers. And as I've mentioned before, restorations do not last forever. If a veneer chips or breaks, it will need to be replaced. I actually do far fewer veneers these days than I did in the past.

CROWNS OR CAPS

Crowns and caps are the same thing, essentially thimbles that cover existing teeth when too much of the structure is missing and veneers no longer work. The materials used for crowns have changed over the years. Initially, they were made of gold, and yellow gold crowns were very popular because they were strong and fit the tooth well.

The downside was their aesthetics. Though in some cultures they are a symbol of power, they just don't look natural—and in the United States, we try to make restorations look as natural as possible, so they blend in with the rest of the mouth. Recently, we have eliminated metal crowns altogether.

In the past, a porcelain coating was bonded to various metals, precious and nonprecious, to make crowns for the most visible teeth. These metals gave the crown strength and the porcelain provided beauty. Nowadays, instead of metal we're using ceramic materials that are extremely strong and look great, eliminating the need for porcelain bonding. They are made with milling machines instead of casting systems, enabling labs and dentists to design restorations digitally, which makes the restorations more accurate than ever.

DENTAL IMPLANTS

There comes a point when a tooth is so decayed or broken that a restoration is no longer possible. In the past, the only choices a dentist had were making a fixed bridge or a partial denture. A fixed bridge was the better way of dealing with the situation. Neighboring teeth were used to support the replacement tooth. The removable partial denture comes in and out of the mouth. It is made of metal and plastic, and provides the most economical way of replacing some missing teeth. The removable denture is not as comfortable as a permanent restoration and does not function as well as your own teeth, but we still do them.

In the past few decades, dentists have been perfecting implants. An implant is made of metal, often a titanium alloy that is embedded into the jaw bone to be used as a post to support a porcelain tooth. Implants can replace a single tooth or a full arch of teeth—though there are some limitations to implant placement. For an implant to be successful, there has to be enough bone to support it. Financial considerations also are an issue. The method is a bit more expensive, but the results are far superior to bridges and partial dentures.

Each of these options—whitening, orthodontics, veneers, crowns, and implants—is an acceptable option for creating a functional, beautiful smile. Each comes with a price, so it is up to you to decide what your smile is worth. Will it help you get a new job? What about a date? My patients who work in the media are required to have a beautiful smile. Not sure what a new smile will look like? We can use cosmetic imaging to give you an idea and help you make a decision about whether to go ahead with a cosmetic procedure.

Back in the day, we used to take a picture and alter it with Photoshop. It's not that difficult. I started a cosmetic imaging center in my office twenty years ago without the aid of digital cameras. I used a large video camera and an elaborate computer system to make this happen. Now everything is easier and the simulations are even better. Ask your dentist to show you what you'd look like with whitening or veneers or even orthodontia. It will make you more comfortable with your decision.

We know it's an investment, but we also know how it changes people's lives. That's what dentists do: We change people's lives. Cosmetic dentistry builds self-esteem and confidence, making you feel better about yourself. Our smiles are the first thing other people see and remember. We try in so many ways to make a good impression, but being unable to smile could negate all other efforts.

> **We know it's an investment, but we also know how it changes people's lives.**

Some of my patients invest in the best clothes and wear beautiful jewelry. They have spent a small fortune on facelifts and liposuction but never have paid much attention to their smiles. Sometimes improving a smile obviates the need to do anything else.

Want to change your life? Take a look in the mirror and then go see your dentist to discuss what can be done to make you feel and look better. That's how you change your life.

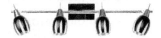

Chapter 9

TEN THINGS YOU NEED TO KNOW ABOUT DENTAL INSURANCE

Before we get into the nitty gritty of what having dental insurance really means, let's talk about some definitions. What do we mean when we talk about the alphabet soup of DSOs, DMOs, DHMOs, and PPOs?

A DSO is a dental-support organization. These groups contract with dental practices and provide business management and support for nonclinical operations. DSOs allow dentists to focus on patients while letting someone else run the business side. A DSO typically sets up a corporation to pay dentists' salaries, and the set-up typically attracts younger dentists who need to gain experience and prefer a salary as they pay off their student loans. Dentists working for DSOs often complain of high-stress environments that make profit a priority over patient care. They are often given quotas each month and have to do a certain number of crowns every week. Among the other downsides is that care that's more complex than basic dentistry needs to be referred out to specialists. DSOs actually own the business. The dentist is an employee and has but little influence in the operation of the practice. The DSO determines what materials are used on patients, what laboratories can be used to fabricate dental prostheses, and all the important decisions dedicated to the bottom line. They have become popular due to economics of scale: The bigger organizations have better buying power with suppliers, and central billing offices cut down duplication in multiple locations. The independent dentist has been turned into a business run by a corporation.

A DMO is a dental maintenance plan. DMOs provide a lower-cost benefit and insurance plan that allows patients to choose a primary-care dentist from a list provided by the insurer. This primary care dentist is responsible for routine care, but if a specialist is needed, the primary-care dentist needs to provide a referral. The plans generally have no deductibles or annual maximums. You might not even have a co-pay. However, you cannot see a dentist or specialist outside the plan without a referral. If you do, you might have to shoulder the entire cost. It's not uncommon to see a different dentist every time you go. Since they have such a large turnover, continuity of care is limited.

A DHMO is a dental health maintenance organization. These plans do not have deductibles or maximums. Instead, you receive service for a fixed dollar amount for a treatment. Often there is no co-pay or just a nominal one for diagnostic and preventive services. The DHMO offices offer extremely low-cost services. Like a DMO, you will need to select your dentist from a list of network providers. These plans provide basic services and are less expensive, but individual needs vary, and some treatments may not be covered at all. Networks also are extremely limited.

A dental PPO is a preferred provider organization. These plans also have networks but offer more balance between lower costs and choice of dentist. You can switch dentists at any time without having to clear it with your insurance company, and there is coverage whether you go to an in-network or out-of-network dentist, although coverage out of network may not be reimbursed at the same rate. In-network dentists have agreed not to charge more than a certain amount for a specific procedure; though the fee for a procedure will be discounted, you will still be responsible for any charges the insurance company does not pick up. If you use an out-of-network provider, that amount can be somewhat higher. Often preventive charges are covered at 100 percent whether in or out of network. Network providers file claims for you, and often out-of-network offices will do the same. Many of these plans also have annual deductibles, the amounts of which vary from plan to plan, and there are annual caps on coverage.

Independent/concierge practices provide services without intervention by insurance companies. They allow dentists to consider patient needs more fully and make decisions on what is needed rather than what insurance will cover. These offices are not controlled by the insurance industry or by large corporations. Independent dentists can run their practices the way they want. This means investing in technology, using high-end laboratories that would be cost-prohibitive for an in-network practice, and having enough staff and equipment to serve their patients better. Also, these practices usually maintain their equipment and offices better than others.

Would you rather have your care determined by an experienced professional with your best interests in mind or a document written by a lawyer and arbitrated by a clerk

Would you rather have your care determined by an experienced professional with your best interests in mind or a document written by a lawyer and arbitrated by a clerk with an eye toward maximizing profits?

with an eye toward maximizing profits? Remember, there are hundreds of different types of plans. Whether they are DMOs or PPOs, they are written so the insurance companies benefit in the long run.

There's also a new wrinkle in this whole insurance business: Some dentists are now offering patients the option of a subscription service that provides many of the benefits of insurance without the middle man.[20] For a monthly fee paid directly to the dentist, patients are guaranteed a discount on services. These monthly fees are much lower than traditional dental-insurance policies. At the same time, the dentist avoids the hassle of filing claims and the office overhead associated with that. These services are only available at the office with which you sign up. They are not transferable, and if you don't use the services for which you are prepaying, you don't get reimbursed.

The bottom line is that over the years, dentists have become trapped in the dental-insurance business, and this has dramatically changed dentistry forever. Dentists initially added these plans to fill holes in their schedules and ended up relying on the insurance companies for their livelihood. Their reimbursement has dropped year after year while expenses have grown. Personalized care has morphed into assembly lines getting patients in and out as fast as possible.

WHAT YOU NEED TO KNOW

There are ten things you need to know about dental insurance:

1. **Insurance companies don't work for you.** They work for their shareholders and want to pay out as little as possible. That means they turn down claims whenever they can. Offices need

---

20 Marcella S. Kreiter, "Pennsylvania Startup Takes the Middleman Out of Dental Costs," *Crain's Philadelphia*, October 10, 2017, http://philadelphia.crains. com/article/news/pennsylvania-startup-takes-middleman-out-dental-costs.

to have full-time staff just to fight with the insurance companies. Carriers also delay payment as long as possible. When they finally pay, it's for the least amount your policy allows. Just because an insurance company says a procedure is not allowed doesn't mean you don't need it. It just means that the policy doesn't cover it, or your employer only included certain types of coverage. You have to trust your doctor when it comes to making decisions about your health. If you don't trust your dentist, you need to find a different one. Your insurance policy might cover two visits a year for your care, while your dentist suggests you come in four times because of your diabetes and periodontal disease. Just because your insurance company won't pay for it does not mean you shouldn't go!

2. **You need to understand how DMOs and DHMOs work.**
A lot of offices don't participate because they're so restrictive, and their reimbursement rates are so low. These plans provide participating dentists a fixed amount per patient, usually about $15 a month. So, if a dentist is handling fifteen hundred patients for a given plan, that's $22,500 a month whether the patients come in for service or not. The incentive here for the dentist is to provide as little treatment as possible to maximize profit. That means just basic dentistry—X-rays and cleanings, easy fillings— not full dental health care. The minute they start doing a lot of work, they're losing money. That's why a lot of offices don't participate in these plans. Patients also find they usually need to wait a long time for an appointment.

3. **If you have a dental PPO, using an out-of-network provider may not be as expensive as you think.**
Surprisingly, preventive procedures like X-rays, cleanings, and

checkups are covered at 80 to 100 percent, even if you go out of network. Other procedures will cost a bit more but it may not be that much, depending on how your policy is written (e.g., whether there's a fee schedule or if payments are based on a percentage). You need to know what's in your policy. Don't expect your dental office to know the ins and outs of your dental plan. There is often fine print that is not accessible to an out-of-network office. Most offices do their best to maximize your benefits, but patients need to take some responsibility by investigating their coverage. Time after time we get complaints about insurance coverage. Dental insurance is not like medical insurance; it is there to help with payment. It is not there to cover all of your bills.

4. **You get what you pay for.** Much of the advertising by corporate dental offices emphasizes low rates. They are treating dentistry like a commodity, a one-size-fits-all service. But it's not. If you need heart surgery, are you going to look for the least expensive surgeon? Probably not. It wouldn't be the smartest thing to do. Going out of network could mean getting more comprehensive care and superior quality for the work performed.

5. **We at Advanced DDS, and other similar independent offices, do not work for the insurance company; and though we do our best, we can't know everything about your coverage.** We will work hard to get the most benefits possible for our patients, but we do not have control over what is covered. Again, there literally are thousands of plans out there. Often, insurance companies won't tell us over the phone how much they're willing to cover, making it tough to come up with numbers. You need to know whether there is a fee schedule or whether the insurance pays a percentage. Be your

own insurance advocate and bring any necessary information with you. Don't expect the dentist to know everything about your coverage.

6. **Cheaper does not mean better.** Look at the bottom of the insurance statement you get. It may include a line saying that staying in network will cost you less. However, it doesn't say staying in network will provide the same or better treatment. There are plenty of good dentists out there, but you get what you pay for. It's expensive to run a dental office, especially with all the new technology out there. If you need to cut corners, where do you start? When a fee schedule is involved, the insurance company likely pays very little toward the treatment, maybe $10 or $15. It may be better than nothing—but it's not going to cover the entire bill. When I started my practice in the 1980s, insurance companies were paying out $1,500 per year to cover patients. Now, they're paying $1,500 to $2,000, despite nearly forty years of inflation and the explosion of technology. The payments don't cover overhead. The insurance companies are playing games here. You need to start thinking of insurance coverage as a supplement rather than something that will take care of all your dental needs.

7. **Insurance companies are reducing dental benefits.** They may not tell you this, but dentists receive notices all the time. One company is dropping its fees 15 percent. Where should the dental office make up that 15 percent? Reduce the time spent with patients? Reduce the quality of materials used for fillings and crowns? Find a less expensive lab to produce its restorations? Somewhere a corner is going to be cut. Just remember that.

8. **Insurance companies try very hard to reject claims.** We'll file a claim, and the insurance company will say they never

received it. We'll file again, and they will say they need more information. We'll send in the additional information, and they will deny the claim and tell the patient to appeal. It's a racket—and it's working against our patients. We try to get as much coverage as possible, but it's not easy.

9. **Quality of care and the experience of the dentists involved are not listed by the insurance companies.** They tell you it's less expensive to stay within their networks, but would you rather see a dentist fresh out of school with less than two years of experience or go to an office where the combined experience of the dentists involved is around eighty years? The examination is the most important part of a routine visit. We want to know if our patients have periodontal disease. We want to know if there are any major cavities. We want to evaluate the bite for occlusion. All these questions need to be answered during an examination. It's *not* irrelevant—and no, not every dentist out there has the experience and expertise to identify problems in the early stages.

10. **Our goal is for you to keep your teeth for a lifetime.** For us to do that, we need to be fairly compensated, and working through insurance does not provide that. Are you willing to work for a fraction of what you deserve? Well, neither should your dentist. Experience, quality materials, and high-end technology all cost money. Your smile is worth it.

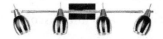

Chapter 10

BABY TEETH ARE MORE IMPORTANT THAN YOU THINK

Think about this: A child's first experience with dental pain comes in infancy. Cutting those first teeth is excruciating. A baby may cry for hours on end, the only relief coming from a frozen teething ring. Mercifully, there's no conscious memory of the experience.

So why do parents dredge up that experience with non-reassuring comments like:

- Don't worry, the dentist won't hurt you.
- They will give you a shot with a big needle. It will be fine.
- They will use a drill on your teeth. You will need to stay still.
- Everybody hates the dentist. It's okay.
- They are going to pull your tooth out.

Comments like these set children up for failure and may color their attitude toward dentists for the rest of their lives.

All too often parents transfer their own fears of the dentist onto their children, sometimes before that very first visit. We see many fearful adults at Advanced DDS and discover that those fears began when they were just children. But dentistry does not have to strike fear in anyone's heart—not even a child's. There are methods for numbing a tooth that yield very little discomfort. Most treatment rooms for children have televisions and video games to keep them occupied. The days when a child was tied down and the mouth was forced open are over. A pedodontist (a dentist who specializes in children) or a highly trained general dentist can make a dental visit, if not a fun experience, at least one that will yield no negative residual effects.

So, what do parents need to know?

KEEP YOUR FEARS TO YOURSELF

First of all, don't set your child up for failure by allowing your own fears to rub off on them. Let the dentist explain what will happen. You can find a children's dentist who is kind and compassionate, somebody who's willing to spend the time it takes to make your child's appointment pleasant. If you think the dentist is being too rough or physical with your child, discuss it, since there are times when the dentist needs to take control.

We decided to hire a pedodontist at Advanced DDS because of demand for such services in this area, and she is just wonderful with children. There are numerous general dentists who treat children, but pedodontists have an extra two years of training as well as expertise in sedation and child development. They're also trained in handling behavioral issues along with disabled and medically compromised children. Pedodontists also treat children as young as a year old, while most general dentists don't feel comfortable until a child is four or five. General dentists are just not equipped to handle all child-related situations.

In some cases, the parent gets in the way of a child's treatment. If a child doesn't want to open his mouth, don't tell him it's okay. This does not help your child or the dentist. Leave the dentist alone to do what needs to be done. Getting involved only makes the treatment more difficult. If you don't trust the dentist with your child, find another dentist. You need this trust or it never will work.

THAT FIRST VISIT

Our pedodontist has a saying: "First tooth, first year, time for the first dental visit." You want the visit to be easy and fun. That first visit should involve just counting and cleaning the teeth. Waiting until there is a cavity, pain, and swelling is not very smart and will create a very difficult visit that is tough to overcome. Prevention is always better than waiting for problems.

Teeth actually begin developing very early. A primitive mouth forms by the third week after conception, followed by the tongue, jaws, and palate. By the sixth week of pregnancy, tooth buds that eventually will produce teeth begin forming, and by eight weeks the baby teeth can be discerned. Believe it or not, tooth buds for the permanent teeth begin to develop by the twentieth week.

Baby teeth begin showing up on the gums' surface at about six months of age. There usually are twenty of them, and they're in by the time a child reaches age two-and-a-half. When these teeth first show up, they're not fully formed. They continue to grow and develop roots. As the child grows, the jaw expands, and the baby teeth develop spaces between them to make room for the permanent teeth, which can show up as early as age five, though they usually begin coming in at age six. The first permanent molars don't make an appearance until age six, followed by a second set of molars at age twelve. There's a third set of molars, the wisdom teeth. Not everyone gets them. For those who do, they may be problematic and need to be removed. It is recommended that a panoramic x-ray be taken at age seventeen to evaluate the eruption of the third molars. Their teeth could be impacted (unable to erupt) or could be coming in at angles. It is best to have these teeth removed before college.

When you look at a young child's x-ray, you'll be amazed at exactly how many teeth are in the mouth. Even the adult molars and wisdom teeth are there, though they won't make an appearance for years. These permanent teeth must be protected for later in life. An easy way to do that is the use of sealants on the baby teeth.

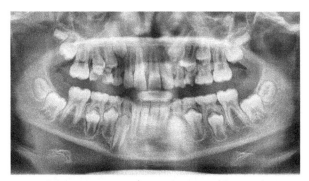

Panoramic x-ray of an eight-year-old's mouth
showing both baby and adult teeth

Teeth have grooves, pits, and fissures on the surface, areas where bacteria can live and cause decay. A dental sealant is a plastic coating that covers the tooth's surface. Such sealants can also be placed on permanent molars, sealing the grooves to prevent bacteria from taking root in the crevices. It's not a panacea for tooth decay, since only the top of the tooth is protected. There are four other surfaces that can rot, so regular checkups are still necessary.

BABY TEETH ARE IMPORTANT

Parents ask me why it's necessary to fix baby teeth, since the child will just lose them in a few years. Some baby teeth can stay in the mouth until a child becomes a teenager. I've seen instances where a person's first primary molars are still in the mouth until the ages of forty or fifty. These teeth have a role in a child's development, not only to chew food but to help with the development of the jaw and other structures.

Baby teeth (the technical term is deciduous teeth) hold the spaces in which the permanent teeth will erupt. What happens if a baby tooth is lost prematurely and the space is not preserved? Other teeth might shift position to fill the space. This is a problem because it will prevent the adult tooth from going where it is supposed to go. Your dentist might recommend a space maintainer to prevent this from happening. That way, when the adult tooth erupts, it has plenty of room. Failure to maintain that space might result in the need for braces later on.

Just as some teeth are lost too early, others can hang on too long, which is why a child's mouth needs to be monitored regularly. A baby tooth that's over retained can prevent an adult tooth from coming in, causing long-term problems. Proper bite or occlusion will not be established and spacing in the mouth will be less than optimal. The adult teeth will be crowded. The mouth is very dynamic, and small problems can lead to a chain reaction resulting in many problems. Eruption of the permanent tooth triggers the resorption process for the root of the baby tooth. When the root disappears, the tooth falls out. But if there's no adult tooth to start the process, the baby tooth will not fall out. It can't. That's when the dentist needs to intervene.

Baby teeth also help with proper speech development and nutrition. Losing front teeth early might result in a speech impediment and the need down the line for speech therapy. If an infection develops around a decayed baby tooth, the permanent tooth below can be damaged, becoming discolored or even malformed.

Baby teeth can decay, sometimes very early in life. We call it nursing-bottle syndrome, which is common in babies who are put down in their cribs with bottles of juice. Parents do this to try to keep the baby quiet at night so they can get some sleep. What they don't realize is the sugar in the juice damages the tooth enamel. They're actually bathing the teeth in sugar. If this is done night after night, the enamel starts to deteriorate as the bacteria, Streptococcus mutans and Lactobacillus, consume the sugar in the juice, creating acids.

Preventing cavities is always better than having to fix them. High-sugar diets, drinks, and snacks are among the most common causes of decay. Overuse of sippy cups and bottles, which a child can use for hours at a time, with sugary drinks, lack of brushing, and non-fluoridated water also contribute. It is not uncommon to see a two-year-old with blackened, rotten teeth. This decay must be treated before all the teeth are lost. Children that young, however, cannot be expected to sit in the dental chair for long.

Pacifiers or even a child's thumb are not the answer either. Though sucking on a pacifier might reduce the risk of sudden infant death syndrome and is an easier habit to break than thumb sucking, it increases the risk of middle ear infections. If one is used, however, it should be taken away at the child's first birthday. The longer a child uses a pacifier, the greater the risk of damage to the teeth, jaw, or bite.[21]

---

21 "Pacifiers: Pros, Cons, and Smart Ways to Use Them," BabyCenter.com, last modified March 2016, https://www.babycenter.com/0_pacifiers-pros-cons-and-smart-ways-to-use-them_128.bc.

CHILDREN AND ANESTHESIA

Very young children who need major dental treatment or those with behavioral problems can be treated with general anesthesia, which requires the presence of an anesthesiologist. I know this seems a bit radical for a two-year-old, but the repercussions of leaving the teeth untreated are far worse.

There are different types of sedation for children. General anesthesia puts them fully to sleep, and they are intubated. This is recommended for children too young to be cooperative. Oral sedation also is an option. The child drinks a solution that causes grogginess. Nitrous oxide is a third option. Both oral sedation and nitrous oxide can be used in conjunction with local anesthetics.

Nitrous oxide works well for simple dental visits. There is a nose piece through which a child breathes. Sometimes these carry a scent that is appealing to the child to make him or her relaxed and cooperative.

When my oldest child was eight, he developed an extra tooth that needed to be removed. It's called a supernumerary tooth, something that is very common. They can develop anywhere in the mouth. This one was between the upper two front teeth. I needed a cooperative patient for the procedure and decided to use nitrous oxide with a local anesthetic. My son's reaction has always stuck with me. He said the nitrous oxide made him feel like he was in a cartoon, and that's how I've described it to children ever since. Nitrous oxide is great for both children and adults, but when it comes to describing the experience for adults, I don't mention cartoons. Instead I tell them it's like having a few glasses of wine.

The opposite of supernumerary teeth would be congenitally missing teeth. Sometimes teeth never have tooth buds and so never develop. The most common teeth to be missing are the upper lateral incisors, the two teeth next to the front teeth, and the lower bicuspids, the double-pointed teeth next to the canines. It's important to determine if the teeth actually are missing or are just late in developing. If they really are missing, there are two options: One is to keep the space open with braces so an implant can be done later in life; the other is to move all the teeth together and position the eye teeth or canines in the lateral position so they can be reshaped later to look like an incisor. Both options work, and it is up to the dentist and parents to determine which is best.

Children should be seen by a dentist every six months, so tooth growth can be monitored, and problems can be treated early. Waiting for pain or obvious holes amounts to neglect. Don't say baby teeth aren't worth saving. They are! The future of your child's permanent teeth is partially dependent on the care given to baby teeth.

Children should be taught proper dental hygiene at an early age. Make sure they brush morning and night to develop a lifetime of good oral habits. Use fluoridated water or fluoride supplements while baby and adult teeth are developing. Following these steps will help your children have a strong, healthy mouth for a lifetime.

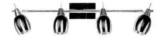

CONCLUSION

I hope I have helped you understand the way you should approach your dental care and the way you should think about your dentist, your mouth, and the question of insurance. I'm here to educate you.

Going to the dentist doesn't have to hurt. You don't have to accept the level of care dictated by your insurance. And most of all, you need to invest in yourself.

I have had new patients come in and say they've never seen an office like Advanced DDS. They've never been treated the way I treat them. They've never seen staff like mine. They've never seen this level of technical know-how and modern equipment. They say they wished they had discovered us ten years earlier.

I wish they had, too, so their dental problems would not be so advanced. It's never cheaper to put off dental work. The longer you wait, the more expensive it gets.

Work on your mouth should be done the right way the first time. It will save you pain and money. And remember, there are options in nearly every instance.

You need to be an advocate for yourself and understand what is going on. And most importantly, you need to trust your dentist. Don't go in blind. When you enter a dental office for the first time, it's never wrong to ask questions. Is the dentist up to date? Does he or she offer the services you really need? If the services are cheap, *why* are they so cheap? Just because insurance pays for something doesn't mean it's the right answer for your needs.

My best patient is the educated patient. People have very little knowledge about not only dentistry in genera, but of the dental industry overall. They have no idea that one office is different from another. They only know the fees are different.

Advanced DDS is a high-end practice. It's by no means the only one. There are other dentists who have made investments in new technology and equipment all over the country, but we're few and far between.

Patients say my office is exactly what they were looking for: clean, state of the art, well run, and friendly. People are grateful we have sedation available. The massage chairs are a nice bonus. Our pedodontist is great with children, making it a fun experience.

I'm not belittling less advanced and less all-encompassing practices. All practices serve a purpose. You just need to decide what's best for you.

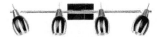

ACKNOWLEDGMENTS

'd like to thank consultant Jay Geier for encouraging me to put on paper what we've been doing for years to improve our dental health. To my wife, Elisa, who has been at my side from day one in practice and has encouraged me to pursue my quest for the best dental practice I could have. And to all the patients I have seen over the years; their trust in me has enabled me to grow my practice and allowed me to help many, many more people.

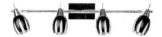

ABOUT THE AUTHOR

D r. Brian Raskin, CEO of Advanced DDS—a progressive group practice that excels in customer service and the most advanced techniques in restoring one's oral health—is a 1982 graduate of New York University College of Dentistry, the same school from which his father and grandfather graduated from in 1953 and 1923, respectively.

Dr. Raskin completed his residency in general practice at Booth Memorial Hospital in 1983, and since then, he has taken more than two thousand hours of continuing education, covering many phases of dentistry. He was trained by Dr. Carl Misch, an expert and major innovator in implant dentistry and the driving force behind Dr. Raskin's mastery of the implant field.

As he's built his practice, Dr. Raskin has found many people put off dental treatment due to fear of pain. Conventional techniques such as nitrous oxide sedation, talking, or trying to reason with a patient were not enough to motivate people to complete needed treatment. So Dr. Raskin took a mini-residency in IV sedation dentistry at Montefiore Hospital in the Bronx, New York. Here, Dr. Raskin learned how to successfully and safely sedate his patients so they could be comfortable and anxiety free while going forward with their needed dentistry.

Dr. Raskin is also a big believer in technology. His office offers the most advanced computer and lab equipment available for a dental practice. These technologies make his patients visits shorter and easier. He feels investing in patients by adding new technology should be mandatory. At Advanced DDS, you will always find the best equipment, technology, and techniques available to a dentist.

Dr. Raskin's office is in Garden City, Long Island, New York.

Contact

Advanced DDS

200 Garden City Plaza STE 101, Garden City, NY 11530

www.advanceddds.com

www.drbrianraskin.com

www.advancedchildrensdentistry.com

To see some of my photography, which has been a passion for most of my life, visit: www.brianraskin.com.

Printed in the USA
CPSIA information can be obtained
at www.ICGtesting.com
JSHW012055140824
68134JS00035B/3461

9 781599 329949